Advance Praise for *This Book Will Save Your Life*

"This is a pointed and urgent challenge not just for those suffering addiction, but for all of us who care about the dignity of the human person and sacredness of human life. Sure, there's a lot of bad news about addiction, but there's a lot of good news as well. My friend Dr. Russell Surasky gives us hope for a culture of recovery."

—Timothy Michael Cardinal Dolan, Archbishop of New York

"The lifesaving information in this book could be your last hope for survival and for those you cherish. Don't wait until it's too late."

—Dr. Drew Pinsky, Celebrity Internist, Addiction Medicine Specialist

THIS BOOK WILL
SAVE YOUR LIFE

THIS BOOK WILL
SAVE YOUR LIFE

The New Medical Cure for Opioid Addiction

Dr. Russell Surasky

Post Hill
PRESS

A POST HILL PRESS BOOK
ISBN: 979-8-88845-625-5
ISBN (eBook): 979-8-88845-626-2

This Book Will Save Your Life:
The New Medical Cure for Opioid Addiction
© 2024 by Dr. Russell Surasky
All Rights Reserved

Cover photo by Barry Morgenstein

This is a work of nonfiction. All people, locations, events, and situations are portrayed to the best of the author's memory.

Post Hill Press
New York • Nashville
posthillpress.com

Published in the United States of America
1 2 3 4 5 6 7 8 9 10

TABLE OF CONTENTS

Foreword.. ix

Introduction xiii

PART I.   UNRAVELING OPIOID ADDICTION AND ITS
           GRIP ON HUMANITY

1. A Neurologist's Mission to Transform the World 3

2. Into the Abyss: The Worst Drug Crisis in
    American History 9

3. Cracking the Code: Why Some Suffer with
    Addiction and Others Do Not 12

4. Demystifying Opioids: What Exactly Are They? 22

5. Fentanyl's Grip on America 31

6. Breakthrough Science: A Tale of Two Brains 34

PART II.   THE EVOLUTION OF MEDICATION-ASSISTED
           TREATMENTS: METHADONE, SUBOXONE,
           AND THE RISE OF VIVITROL

7. Methadone and Suboxone Unmasked 43

8. Vivitrol: Revolutionizing Addiction Treatment 51

9. Silencing the Savior: The Forces Blocking
    Vivitrol's Revelation 61
10. Vivitrol: Frequently Asked Questions.................................67

PART III. PATHWAYS TO RECOVERY: 12-STEP SUCCESS,
          RELAPSE RESILIENCE, AND SUSTAINED
          SOBRIETY

11. Lost in the Maze: Navigating the Complex
    World of Addiction Treatment Programs...........................83
12. The Science Behind 12-Step Programs 87
13. Integrating Holistic Treatments in Addiction Recovery 96
14. Relapse: The Greatest Teacher of All...................................102
15. Sustaining Sobriety: Practical Strategies for
    Long-Term Recovery 107

PART IV. BEYOND BOUNDARIES: TRANSFORMING
         PERSPECTIVES, STRENGTHENING FAMILIES,
         AND EMBRACING TELEMEDICINE IN
         ADDICTION CARE

16. Shattering the Stigma of Addiction......................117
17. Addiction Is a Family Disease 124
18. Recovery Crossroads: Navigating Marijuana's
    Role in Sobriety 133
19. Telemedicine: The New Frontier 140
20. The Blueprint for Healing 144
References 147
About the Author..153

FOREWORD

I f you, a family member, or someone you love is struggling with addiction (substance use disorder, or SUD), it's normal to feel overwhelmed and desperate. Left untreated, addiction is a progressive and deadly illness. You may also start to understand that your ability to help is somewhat limited. If it's you who is manifesting features of this condition, the lack of clarity around solutions is no doubt adding to your sense of desperation. Trying to get help for a SUD, or attempting to find help for someone you love, can feel desperate and overwhelming. No doubt adding to your anguish is the buzzing, blooming landscape of addiction treatments and confusing, conflicting sources of information.

As a medical doctor and addictionologist for over thirty years, I can tell you beyond any shadow of a doubt that addiction is a neurological brain disease and not a behavioral or psychological condition. Addiction is a complex medical illness and therefore it's critical to have a specialized physician perform the evaluation and treatment. Additionally, those suffering from SUD often have psychiatric and medical concomitant disorders that also require diagnosis and treatment by skilled practitioners. Medical doctors often require years of experience treating these types of patients before they can develop such expertise. Unfortunately, very few physicians are fully and adequately trained to manage these disorders.

As a physician with decades of experience in the field of addiction medicine, I can tell you how incredibly rare it is to meet another doctor with the requisite level of expertise and experience that's truly required. Dr. Russell Surasky, a double board-certified neurologist, is such a physician. Dr. Surasky and I are in complete alignment with our perspective and philosophy, and he has my unequivocal support.

The information you are about to learn from this book will change everything you thought you knew about addiction and its treatment. You will come to understand the newest science showing us that addiction is caused by the hijacking or "rewiring" of key regions in the brain. Most importantly, you will learn about groundbreaking medicine that can save your life and the lives of those you love the most. This book just may turn the tide on this entire pandemic, saving countless lives and easing untold amounts of suffering.

Even with these new incredible medication-based protocols, studies show us that it's medication + counseling that provides the best chance at sustained sobriety. Counseling can come in many forms, but it has been my experience that 12-step meetings (mutual aid societies) are enormously impactful. I have been working in a psychiatric hospital since 1985, and I administered an inpatient chemical dependency program from 1991 to 2010. I have seen many trends and ideas come and go in the field of addiction treatment. Twelve-step/mutual aid societies have always remained a constant in the treatment world. The evidence for their effectiveness is now overwhelming. Recent studies out of Harvard University indicate that a 12-step program is as efficacious, or more so, than any other professionally managed form of counseling. In a time of restricted resources, it makes no sense to undermine a treatment that stands up to scientific scrutiny and is *free*. And the system of mutual aid creates people who readily offer manpower to help out, just as they themselves were helped during their time of need. Dr. Surasky and I have discussed this subject on many occasions, and we are in complete alignment! I was thrilled to see that Dr. Surasky, in addition to teaching you about new and remarkable medication protocols, has also dedicated a part of this book to helping you understand the science and power behind 12-step meetings.

Today, there are many new and exciting approaches to the neurobiology of addiction. In this book, Dr. Surasky not only fully explains the neurological brain changes that cause addiction but also lays out a never-before-seen medication protocol that will likely change the way we treat addiction in this country. This is a handbook that will offer you tremendous hope and alleviate your sense of desperation as you come to learn that no matter what the situation, recovery is always possible.

—**Drew Pinsky, MD (Dr. Drew)**

INTRODUCTION

Before you start reading chapter 1, I want you to know that the book you're holding in your hands contains the answers that can save your life, the life of a loved one, or if you're a doctor—the life of your patient.

I want to start by telling you a story about a young man named Travis. Just seventeen years old at the time, Travis had everything going for him. He was handsome, exceedingly bright, and the most compassionate person I knew. He had incredibly loving and supportive parents and was always surrounded by wonderful friends. One day, during a particularly competitive lacrosse match, a player on the opposite team hit Travis in the face with their lacrosse stick. Having personally witnessed this incident, I can attest to just how much pain Travis must have been feeling. What struck me the most was just how forgiving Travis was toward the player who had hurt him. While Travis's teammates were on the verge of fighting with the other team, he repeatedly insisted that they stop and kept reminding everyone that "it was just an accident." Due to his injury, Travis could no longer play lacrosse during his senior year and ultimately required extensive orthopedic surgery to correct his jaw. The procedure went smoothly but after the surgery, an unforeseen problem emerged.

"Oh my God," he told me when I visited him in the hospital, "this medication is amazing." The hospital had administered intravenous Dilaudid (a brand name of hydromorphone) to Travis, an extraordinarily powerful and addictive opioid. Hospitals often use it for post-operative patients because it's fast-acting and manages pain well. But for Travis, it did more than manage his physical pain. It gave him a sense of euphoria.

When I spent time with Travis a few weeks after his surgery, I saw several pill bottles in his room, all containing opiate pain medicines. I was not a physician at the time and just assumed that he was taking the necessary medicines that were prescribed by his doctor.

Shortly after his surgery, Travis went off to college as planned. This was at the same time that I was entering medical school. We were now living in different states from each other, and I had stopped hearing from him as much. What I didn't know at the time was that once his doctors had stopped prescribing him pain medicine, he had instead turned to buying it from people at college. When I did get to speak with him over the phone, I noticed he didn't sound right, not at all like himself. Then it finally dawned on me: "I wonder if he had developed an addiction to those painkillers?"

His parents and I did whatever we could think of to get him the help he needed, including detox, inpatient programs, and numerous outpatient treatment programs. Travis desperately wanted to overcome this opiate addiction and fought extremely hard every step of the way. This time in his life was marked by periods of sobriety as well as frequent relapses. Even while facing these struggles, Travis managed to obtain a bachelor's degree from Indiana University and later a master's degree in social work from Adelphi University in New York. Immediately following graduation, Travis accepted a full-time position at a prestigious facility. He voluntarily took on the role of providing counseling services to those who were struggling with drug and alcohol addiction.

For over ten years, Travis battled his own addiction, but as is so often the case, recovery never seemed to stick. It was as if his addiction refused to let go of him. A short time after he started his new job, the one where he planned to make a positive impact on the lives of those around him, Travis relapsed. Only this time, the pills had been mixed with an even more powerful opioid than oxycodone, called fentanyl. This caused Travis to die of asphyxiation while sleeping at his parents' home.

This was my home. Our home. Travis was my brother.

I've never shared my personal story before, not with my patients or even my closest colleagues. As a doctor, as a neurologist specializing in addiction medicine, I have spent many years speaking and teaching at medical conferences across the country. I'm one of the only doctors in the entire United States who is double board-certified in both neurology and addiction medicine. Additionally, I make regular appearances on national news networks, including several interviews with Tucker Carlson and other well-known news anchors. And yet this is the very first time that I've ever revealed this story about my brother Travis.

Two hundred people in the United States die each day from drug overdoses.[1] In the time it takes you to read this page, another person will have died. I wrote this book for Travis and the nearly 250 million others in the world who are struggling with addiction at this very moment. It's critical to realize that there are very few illnesses that can destroy a life as fast as opiate addiction. It wreaks havoc on everything from brain cells to social bonds, leaving lives destroyed—and families, along with communities, shattered—in its devastating wake. Those afflicted experience intense cravings that hijack their lives, leaving family and friends, sons and daughters, fathers and mothers, and brothers and sisters disoriented and lost. While they continue to chase the drug, their family continues to chase them. Addiction causes extreme suffering to both the person who Is addicted and to their entire family. This is why addiction is often accurately described as a family disease. Over just the past couple of years, we have made groundbreaking advancements in our understanding of addiction: exactly where it's occurring in the brain and how we can help save those who are suffering from what's always a life-or-death situation. The information you are about to read comes with great responsibility, as you will possess knowledge that so few others have ever been exposed to. If you are a doctor, you need now what I give you. Out there in those great open spaces are multitudes seeking what you will possess. The burdens are heavy, responsibilities are many, and obligations are providential. But the satisfaction of relieving suf-

---

[1]   Centers for Disease Control and Prevention (CDC). "Provisional Drug Overdose Death Counts." https://www.cdc.gov/nchs/nvss/vsrr/drug-overdose-data.htm#:~:text=1%3B%20natural%20and%20semisynthetic%20opioids,4%3B%20cocaine%2C%20T40.

fering and adding millions of years to the lives of millions of suffering people will bring forth satisfaction and glory with greater blessings than you think. Time is of the essence.

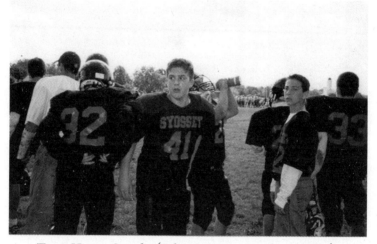

Travis Hunter Surasky (July 18, 1986 – October 3, 2018). My only brother and greatest inspiration. My love for him is eternal. In the beauty of his life and the pain of his struggles, I found the strength and purpose to save others. His journey continues as a beacon of hope for those still fighting.

PART I

UNRAVELING OPIOID ADDICTION AND ITS GRIP ON HUMANITY

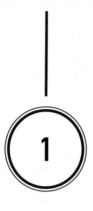

A NEUROLOGIST'S MISSION TO TRANSFORM THE WORLD

The United States of America is now facing the worst drug addiction crisis in its history. Death from drug overdoses now surpasses fatalities from both car crashes and gun violence combined. This means that by the time you finish reading this chapter, another life will have been lost. In just the past few years, fentanyl, an extremely potent and devastatingly harmful opioid, has dramatically altered the landscape of drug addiction and overdoses, unlike any other substance in history. With fentanyl the danger has escalated to a point where virtually anyone is vulnerable, not just those with addiction. Ingesting just one tiny granule of fentanyl powder is enough to kill someone in just a matter of moments. Addiction to drugs, specifically opiate painkillers, was declared a nationwide public health emergency by President Donald Trump in October 2017. In addition, our current president, Joe Biden, has openly discussed his son Hunter's struggles with addiction. While Trump's emergency declaration has increased governmental funding and improved access to treatment—and President Biden's frankness on the topic has helped end some of the stigma around addiction—the epidemic continues to worsen.

We are now at the point where every individual is just one degree of separation from the scourge of addiction. Meaning, if you don't personally suffer from addiction, then it's likely someone very close to you is. Opioid overdose deaths cut across all demographic lines, affecting individuals of all ages, races, and socioeconomic backgrounds. Last year, there were approximately ninety thousand opioid overdose deaths in this country alone. More than forty-eight million Americans are currently suffering from addiction and less than 1 percent of them are getting any type of treatment. Behind the statistics lie the stories of individuals whose lives have been tragically cut short by opioid overdoses. These are sons and daughters, parents and siblings, friends and neighbors whose deaths could have been prevented. Opioid addiction not only exacts a heavy toll on the individual struggling with substance use disorder but also reverberates through their communities, leaving a trail of devastation in its wake.

Approximately 20 percent of the population has battled addiction to drugs or alcohol. Consequently, it's common for hospitalized patients, regardless of their medical issue, to exhibit symptoms of their addiction during their stay. These symptoms range from strong cravings for drugs to severe withdrawal symptoms. Medical students are trained to be vigilant for such signs in all hospitalized patients, irrespective of the primary reason for their admission.

During my medical training as a neurology resident, nearly 100 percent of my time was spent seeing emergency cases in the hospital. Our weeks often extended beyond one hundred hours, with frequent overnight shifts on twenty-four-hour call. As part of my training, I was responsible for managing all emergency stroke cases that arrived at the hospital.

A stroke happens when the brain is deprived of oxygen due to either blocked arteries or brain bleeding. Depending on the location within the brain, strokes can lead to severe and lasting effects such as speech loss, paralysis, and even death. Because of this, immediate intervention by neurologists as soon as the patient enters the emergency room with a stroke is crucial to preserve brain tissue and minimize damage to the brain.

When a stroke patient arrived in the emergency room, a "stroke code" would activate, prompting my pager to sound and requiring me to rush to the emergency department. It wasn't unusual for me to handle over ten emergency stroke cases during each shift. As a neurology resident, my main responsibility was to conduct urgent neurological examinations to identify the location of the stroke in the brain. At the same time, the patient underwent a CT scan of their brain to assess for any bleeding. If they were eligible, I would administer a life-saving clot-dissolving drug called a tissue plasminogen activator (tPA). Several criteria were evaluated in order to determine whether a patient could receive tPA, with one of the most critical being that treatment must be administered within 4.5 hours of the stroke's onset.

I'll always remember a particular night on call at the hospital. Around 3:30 a.m., my pager went off for a stroke emergency in the ER. The patient, aged thirty-eight, had suffered a stroke in the left hemisphere of the brain due to a blockage of the left middle cerebral artery—a common occurrence. Unfortunately, since the stroke had occurred about six hours earlier, he wasn't eligible for tPA treatment.

Initially, the case appeared routine. However, during my patient rounds the next morning, I observed something peculiar. Despite being a heavy smoker for thirty years, the patient declined the nicotine patch I had prescribed. This was surprising, as nicotine cravings and withdrawal can be intense, often prompting patients to feel extremely uncomfortable. I've witnessed cases where patients have refused medical care and left the hospital just to smoke a cigarette. So, when he told the nurse he didn't want the nicotine patch, it was highly unusual. What made it even more unusual was that he continued to refuse the nicotine patch for several days during his hospital stay, without reporting any cravings to smoke. Upon reviewing the patient's brain MRI, I noticed he suffered damage to the insula, a brain region not commonly affected by strokes. This led me to speculate whether the stroke's impact on the insula was linked to the patient's sudden lack of interest in smoking. The insula is a complex brain structure that plays a crucial role in sensory and emotional processing, including pain perception.

Recalling a study I had encountered during my medical school years, I learned that individuals with addiction exhibited increased insular activity when exposed to drug cues, such as scenes depicting drug use in movies. Intrigued, I delved further into related research and discovered a study conducted by the National Institute on Drug Abuse and the National Institute of Neurological Disorders. This study focused on stroke patients with varying patterns of brain injury. Remarkably, in the majority of stroke cases where damage occurred to the insula, patients ceased smoking abruptly and effortlessly. This revelation was an epiphany for me! While I had always understood addiction as a neurological condition rather than a mere "personality weakness" or moral failing, this finding solidified this understanding and brought it to the forefront of my mind.

It is critical to understand that addiction is a neurological brain condition and not a psychological or behavioral problem. Many people incorrectly assume that addiction is caused by someone's "lack of willpower," a moral weakness, or even a mental illness. These false assumptions lead many to believe that addiction treatment should come from a therapist or psychologist rather than from a medical doctor. To the contrary, there has been a recent explosion of science conclusively demonstrating that *addiction is a neurological disease, not a mental health problem.* Our understanding of addiction has grown astronomically in just the last few years. Through advanced brain imaging, including functional MRIs, we have discovered exactly *how opiate drugs and alcohol hijack the brain.* As you will read later in more detail, the limbic system is a critical set of structures located deep within the brain stem, and it is here where the addiction switch is located. It is the limbic system that is vulnerable to being hijacked by drugs and alcohol. Once this hijacking occurs, and the switch of addiction is turned on, it will create a life filled with intense, obsessive drug cravings, often leading to relapse and, too often, death.

Developing addiction is not just about the drug itself; surprisingly, it's more about your brain's specific chemistry and how the two interact. Therefore, it's critical to understand that one's susceptibility toward addiction is highly determined by the genetics of their brain structure. Haven't you ever wondered why a recovering alcoholic is unable to have a single drink, even after many years of complete sobriety? It's not because they have weak morals! For some people, a single exposure to an opioid drug or a drink of alcohol can cause a devastating neurological cascade in the brain—flipping on the switch of addiction. We know beyond any shadow of a doubt that our genetics play an enormous role in determining our susceptibility toward developing addiction. The genetics of addiction are complex, but by the end of this book, you'll understand everything you need to know.

INTO THE ABYSS: THE WORST DRUG CRISIS IN AMERICAN HISTORY

How did we arrive at the deadliest health crisis in American history? The primary villain in this horrifying story was Purdue Pharma, a pharmaceutical company. Purdue created the opioid drug called OxyContin in 1996, and then they trained a salesforce to intentionally mislead doctors. Purdue's goal was to manipulate doctors into prescribing OxyContin to as many Americans as possible. But why would physicians actually go along with this? Some doctors were secretly paid high sums of money to keep prescribing this addictive drug. This, of course, is illegal, so Purdue pretended that they were paying these doctors to take part in speaking engagements that never actually took place. Other doctors prescribed excessive amounts of OxyContin because it caused their patients to become dependent on the drug, meaning if they tried to stop, they would experience horrible withdrawal symptoms. This essentially guaranteed that their patients would need to keep coming back for visits in order to get their OxyContin refilled. It's important to note, however, that not all doctors who prescribed OxyContin had bad intentions. Many physicians were genuinely trying to help their patients and did not fully realize just how highly addictive the drug truly was.

Purdue's marketing department realized that if they could get doctors to prescribe OxyContin not just for cancer-related pain but also for everyday aches and pains, like arthritis or headaches, the company's profits would skyrocket. In order to convince well-meaning doctors to go along with this, Purdue created a massive, fraudulent campaign in which they downplayed OxyContin's addiction risk. The company sent thousands of marketers into doctors' private offices to tell them that OxyContin was far less addictive than the other opioid drugs on the market. The truth is that one OxyContin pill had an effect on the body that lasted double the time as most other opioid medications. Purdue's reps told doctors that this longer duration of action made the medication less addictive, and that they should feel comfortable prescribing it to virtually all of their patients who had pain. Despite there being no evidence to support this claim, most doctors just accepted it as truth. In 2001, Purdue spent nearly $200 million just on marketing and promoting their drug. Their sales pitch worked! In just a few years, doctors were writing six million prescriptions of OxyContin per year! During that same time period, addiction rates skyrocketed, causing immense suffering and countless overdose deaths.

Purdue had unleashed a terribly addictive and dangerous drug on the American public. Lawsuits against Purdue Pharma began to mount across the country, largely from parents whose children died from overdosing on the powerful opioid. By 2019, nearly every state in America was suing Purdue for a combined $2 trillion. Additionally, Purdue pled guilty in federal court to three felony charges for its role in creating the nation's opioid crisis. The company ultimately admitted that it misbranded OxyContin with the intent to defraud and mislead the public. In addition, they pled guilty to charges including conspiracy to defraud the United States and conspiracy to violate the federal Anti-Kickback Statute (paying doctors to prescribe OxyContin). In the end, Purdue wound up paying $8 billion and was forced into bankruptcy.

CRACKING THE CODE: WHY SOME SUFFER WITH ADDICTION AND OTHERS DO NOT

Is Addiction a Disease?

The American Society of Addiction Medicine characterizes addiction as a "chronic relapsing brain disease," necessitating continuous treatment comparable to other medical conditions such as hypertension and diabetes. Our latest neurological research utilizing cutting-edge technology has confirmed that addiction is a progressive brain illness and not just a behavioral condition. As you will come to learn, addiction is a horrific disease that hijacks very specific circuitry within our brains. More specifically, addiction causes alterations in the brain's mesolimbic dopamine pathway, also known as the reward circuitry of the brain. The mesolimbic dopamine pathway is a neural circuit that begins in the brainstem and extends its projections into various critical regions of the brain associated with experiencing pleasure and maintaining motivation in our daily lives. Scientists are now able to visualize these specific regions of the brain that are hijacked by addiction through the use of advanced imaging studies called position-emission tomography (PET) scans. PET scans definitively show that addiction affects the brain circuits involved in reward, motivation, memory, and even inhibitory control. It's important to note that more accurate terminology for the word "addiction" is now "substance use disorder," or SUD, as mentioned in the foreword. For example, someone might be diagnosed with opioid use disorder or alcohol use disorder. Throughout this book you will see the terms "addiction" and "opioid use disorder" used interchangeably.

Unfortunately, despite all of this conclusive evidence, there is still a staggering percentage of the population who believe that addiction is not a disease. Their argument is often based on the premise that people with addiction can choose to stop using drugs. However, this is a highly illogical position to take because simply having free will to make different choices does not disqualify a medical condition from being a disease. The truth is that a significant number of common diseases involve the element of choice: diabetes, hypertension, strokes, heart attacks, etc. These diseases are highly linked to lifestyle choices, and yet the word "disease" is easily accepted here. If a diabetic chooses to exercise, lose weight, and stay away from sugar, his condition will not worsen and can even improve. The same applies to a hypertensive individual who steers clear of certain foods and salt, etc.

But changing lifestyles can be difficult, which is why so many people continue to eat the wrong foods or smoke—or fail to get regular exercise and sleep—even though it worsens their disease process. The bottom line is that having the potential to choose to quit using an addictive drug doesn't mean addiction isn't a disease.

Addiction, like most other diseases, occurs due to a combination of genetic susceptibility along with environmental exposure. In other words, if an individual with a genetic vulnerability toward addiction exposes their brain repeatedly to a particular drug, a devastating neurological cascade will take place in their brain. Once their brain circuitry has been hijacked, that individual will suffer intense compulsions to continue to use the drug, despite recurring harm in their life. Without treatment, addiction is a progressive illness, often leading to death.

Beyond "Free Will"

During decision-making, there is communication between the frontal cortex, known as the conscious or thinking brain, and the limbic system, often referred to as the unconscious or automatic brain. The limbic system of our brain developed millions of years ago and is located in the brain stem. This region of our brain has incredible power over what we feel motivated to do each day. The limbic system is in charge of our survival drives, such as hunger and sexual attraction. Additionally, the limbic system is part of our autonomic nervous system, which helps to run all of our hormones and organ systems. Nature did not leave these critical functions for our "thinking" brain to control. Consider this question—do you "know" how to manage the function of your heart, lungs, or kidneys? Of course not! Not only that, but no matter how hard you tried, you would be unable to interrupt your limbic system's management of your organ systems. This example should demonstrate to you just how much your brain controls without your conscious awareness.

Think about it—nature didn't want our survival drives like hunger or procreation to be left to our thinking brain—because then we could forget! For example, the reason you feel hungry multiple times each day is that the limbic region of your brain, responsible for unconscious processes, sends powerful signals to the cortical region, the seat of conscious thought, essentially forcing you to go and find food. If you try to use the thinking brain to ignore those signals, you will grow more and more uncomfortable until you finally give in and eat. This shows that your limbic brain is far more powerful than your rational brain.

Having the capacity to make the right choices, however, requires that both of these brain systems (the cortex and the limbic system) are functioning properly. If the limbic system of your brain has been hijacked by drugs, you have extraordinarily powerful compulsions to seek out and continue using that drug even if it's destroying your life. In layman's terms, when addiction has taken hold of the limbic system, the "go" button (limbic region) is on full throttle, and the "brake" button (frontal-cortical region) is not strong enough to stop it.

Didn't you ever wonder why those without an addiction to alcohol can have a few sips of wine at a party, put down the glass, and possibly forget about it? Since alcohol doesn't hijack their limbic system, having one drink and stopping is quite easy! An alcoholic could never do this! Why? Because when alcohol enters their brain, it hacks into the subconscious circuitry in the limbic system. The limbic system then screams at the thinking part of the brain to drink more alcohol. Their so-called free will becomes immensely overpowered by their limbic brain. This makes staying away from alcohol, particularly after having one drink, extremely difficult. This is the same concept with someone who is suffering from opioid addiction.

For individuals grappling with opioid addiction, their main focus in life revolves around obtaining opioids like oxycodone, heroin, and fentanyl on a daily basis. This compulsion is so incredibly powerful that the drug use will continue at the expense of all else. Those in the throes of active opioid addiction will often continue to use these drugs despite becoming broke, stealing from friends/family, being arrested, and even living on the streets. Most will lose a tremendous amount of weight because they stop caring about even basic survival drives, such as eating. Look at the drunk man lying on the park bench in the freezing cold, continuing to drink. Many of these people have warm homes and loving families, yet alcohol changes their brain in such a way that all they care about is having more alcohol. Their most basic, primitive desires fade away as the chemically hijacked brain seeks out one source of pleasure—the drug. Individuals who formerly had successful, thriving jobs and loving families now live with one desire: to find more drugs every day. That's why a recovering alcoholic with twenty years of sobriety can take one sip of a glass of wine, and their habitual drinking starts again. Free will plays a part in preventing the recovering alcoholic from taking that first sip. However, once he takes one drink, that tiny sip reignites the limbic area of the brain, triggering the compulsion. The result: their whole life goes off the rails. It's critical to remember that the hijacked unconscious limbic system is the driving force behind an individual's ongoing drug use, often leaving the conscious, thinking part of the brain relatively powerless to intervene.

Genetic Susceptibilities

We all have genetic susceptibilities that make us vulnerable to both physical and mental illnesses. Our degree of vulnerability for any given condition lies on a spectrum, from very low to extremely high risk. It's your genetics combined with your environmental exposure that determines your health. For example, your genetics may put you at high risk of developing addiction, but if you never use drugs or alcohol, then the switch of addiction will never get turned on. Mental health conditions such as schizophrenia, bipolar disorder, and anxiety disorders, as well as medical conditions such as cancer, diabetes, and hypertension, all start with some degree of genetic susceptibility.

Our individual degree of genetic susceptibility toward developing addiction works in exactly the same way. For example, some people are born with a high degree of genetic vulnerability toward addiction. In these individuals, even a small exposure to a particular drug can cause the limbic system of their brain to get hijacked, causing the switch of addiction to turn on. Similarly, if one has a very low degree of genetic susceptibility toward addiction, it's likely that one could drink alcohol or even abuse drugs recreationally and yet never develop addiction. In other words, those with a very low degree of genetic susceptibility toward addiction would need to be exposed to that drug in high degrees for extended periods of time for addiction to occur. It's important to remember that just because your parents don't have a history of addiction doesn't guarantee that you won't either. Genetic vulnerability toward addiction is highly complex and is made up of many genes, sometimes even skipping generations. In other words, even two parents without any history of addiction can have a child who is at high risk.

Additionally, we know that you could have a genetic vulnerability toward certain specific drugs and not others. This is why some individuals have spent many years drinking alcohol responsibly only to develop a deadly opiate addiction after they were prescribed Percocet by the dentist.

Co-occurring Mental Health Disorders

If you experience mental health conditions like depression, anxiety, ADHD (attention deficit hyperactivity disorder), or bipolar disorder, your chances of developing addiction significantly increase. It's still unclear why these issues commonly coincide, but research suggests a strong link. Studies indicate that individuals with one or more mental health conditions are at a much higher risk of developing drug or alcohol addiction compared to those without such conditions.

Based on numerous studies, as well as my clinical experience, it is my strong belief that ADHD confers the greatest risk for developing addiction. ADHD is a real neurological condition that affects close to 8 percent of the world's population. Studies consistently indicate that individuals with ADHD are at a heightened risk of developing addiction compared to those without the condition. Research suggests that the impulsivity, risk-taking behavior, and difficulty with self-regulation commonly seen in ADHD contribute to this increased vulnerability to addiction. Additionally, individuals with ADHD may turn to substances or addictive behaviors as a way to self-medicate or cope with the challenges associated with their condition.

Untreated ADHD greatly increases impulsive behaviors— "jump first and think later." In other words, the impulse to act is faster than the thought process that might stop or change the action. In a recent study using advanced brain imaging techniques like MRI, researchers discovered significant differences in key brain structures among individuals with ADHD, such as the thalamus and the amygdala. These brain changes are thought to be the main reason behind the increased impulsivity associated with ADHD. The thalamus sends messages to the prefrontal cortex (our thinking brain), which is the region responsible for decision-making. When this message signaling doesn't work properly, executive functions, such as impulse control, can lag. Studies also show that untreated ADHD leads to significant problems, including difficulty maintaining jobs, higher rates of divorce, more frequent car accidents, and increased drug use. Individuals with untreated ADHD have much higher rates of developing drug addiction if they aren't properly treated.

A high percentage of parents initially decline medication to address their child's ADHD. It's entirely understandable to hesitate before introducing any medication for your child. However, in nearly all cases, medication eventually becomes part of the treatment plan. Regrettably, this often happens only after the symptoms of ADHD have already caused notable academic and social difficulties. One concern I often hear from parents is whether starting medication in elementary or middle school will make children more willing to try dangerous drugs in high school and college. Numerous medical studies have demonstrated the exact opposite! In fact, studies have shown that by withholding treatment for ADHD, parents dramatically increase the risk that their child will engage in impulsive, risky, and dangerous behavior, including addictive drug use. Indeed, a recent study revealed that children with untreated ADHD face twice the risk of developing addiction compared to those who receive medication for their ADHD. Another study looked at the brain size of teenagers with ADHD who were either taking medication or not. They found big differences between the two groups. The untreated teenagers had less white matter in their brains compared to those without ADHD. Scientists think that the medication helps protect the brain by improving things like myelination, dendritic branching, and spine length. Basically, treating ADHD with medication might help the brain in ways that make it less likely for someone to develop substance use problems.

Adolescence and the Disease of Addiction

The age at which individuals begin using substances is a key factor in determining the likelihood of developing addiction. For instance, a study tracking individuals who started drinking at age twelve found that 15 percent of them developed addiction. In contrast, those who waited until age nineteen had a significantly lower addiction rate of approximately 1 percent. That is a massive difference, but it is not only for alcohol—it's also true for cigarettes and more dangerous drugs, such as opioids. The timing of drug initiation significantly influences the likelihood of addiction due to the ongoing development of the prefrontal cortex, a critical region of the brain responsible for decision-making and impulse control, which continues until approximately age twenty-three. Engaging in drug experimentation before this stage may render the brain's circuitry more susceptible to disruption or alteration, increasing the risk of addiction. Put simply, for those under the age of twenty-three, you have a reactive limbic system (the gas pedal) without the fully developed cortex (the brake pedal).

DEMYSTIFYING OPIOIDS: WHAT EXACTLY ARE THEY?

Despite the opioid crisis impacting nearly every segment of the American populace, most people still understand very little about "opiates" or "opioids." While many in the press and even the majority of medical professionals continue to use the terms "opiates" and "opioids" interchangeably, you should be aware that they are not exactly the same. The term *opiates* technically refers to any drug naturally derived from the opium poppy plant, such as heroin, morphine, and codeine. *Opioids*, on the other hand, are chemical compounds that are "made in the lab" or "synthesized." Opioids include most of the well-known prescription painkillers, such as hydrocodone (e.g., Vicodin), oxycodone (e.g., OxyContin, Percocet), and fentanyl. It's not necessary for you to memorize which painkillers are in the *opiate* family versus which drugs are in the *opioid family* because both groups of painkillers have the same impact on the brain and are equally likely to cause addiction. Because this is a distinction without an important difference, it is generally acceptable to use either term. Throughout this book you will see the words "opioids" and "opiates" used interchangeably.

All of these drugs were primarily designed to help relieve severe pain, and they do this job very effectively. They also play an enormous role in the way we feel mentally and emotionally. For most people, even without a susceptibility toward addiction, they induce feelings of "well-being" and significantly reduce symptoms such as depression and anxiety. Despite these pleasurable feelings, the majority of people are still easily able to take a short course from their doctor and have no trouble stopping them. However, if you were to have a genetic susceptibility toward opiate addiction, then even just a few doses can hijack the brain and flip on the switch of addiction. Frightening statistics show us that up to 20 percent of the population may have some degree of genetic predisposition toward opiate addiction. As you will learn in more detail, drugs of addiction hijack our brain's natural opiate reward system. These drugs bind to our endogenous opiate receptors and cause an incredibly high spike of dopamine, far greater than any natural experience could produce. When our brain "sees" this extraordinary amount of dopamine being released, it then subconsciously determines that the primary drive of life should be to find more of this drug, even at the expense of everything else. It is at this moment that the switch of addiction has been turned on.

Heroin

There has been a long-standing misconception regarding heroin and commonly prescribed opioid pain medicines such as oxycodone or hydrocodone. The common misconception is that heroin is more addictive and dangerous than prescription opioid pills; however, this simply isn't true. First, with regard to their ability to trigger addiction, both heroin and prescription opiate medicines are equally capable of causing the switch of addiction to turn on in the brain. Another common misunderstanding is that if someone takes opiate pills from the street rather than uses heroin, they are then less likely to overdose and die. This thought process is rooted in the misconception that heroin is laced with other deadly opiate drugs, like fentanyl, while the pills are not. The fact is, however, that at this point in time over 90 percent of prescription opiate pills on the street labeled as oxycodone are actually a combination of heroin and/or fentanyl. Drug dealers make these fake oxycodone pills using machines that press together different drugs into the shape of a real oxycodone pill. These fake tablets look exactly as if they came from a prescription bottle, containing even the correct numbers/letters on the surface of the pills. Virtually 100 percent of patients who come to me for opiate addiction treatment have fentanyl in their urine testing. Many of these individuals had no idea that they had been ingesting fentanyl. Always assume that any opioid pill purchased on the street is inauthentic and that there is an extremely high likelihood that it has been mixed with fentanyl. The bottom line is: heroin and prescription opioid pain pills, such as oxycodone, are nearly identical in terms of how they impact the brain. For people with a brain that is susceptible to addiction, taking any opiate can set in motion a devastating neurological cascade that leads to lifelong drug cravings, immense suffering, and, in many cases, death. According to the American Medical Association, up to 20 percent of the general population that is exposed to prescription opiates—even a short supply from the dentist—will then develop brain changes that lead to opiate addiction.[2]

Fentanyl

Over the past couple of years, the drug fentanyl has become a household word.

You've probably seen or heard about fentanyl on the news, as it has become responsible for more overdose deaths than any other drug. Fentanyl is one of the most powerful opioid drugs in the world. In fact, It's fifty to one hundred times more potent than heroin. Fentanyl accounts for the largest number of overdose deaths nationwide, according to the US Centers for Disease Control and Prevention (CDC). The rate of drug overdoses involving this powerful synthetic opioid skyrocketed by 1,600 percent from 2016 to 2022, replacing heroin as the deadliest drug in the United States.

Fentanyl is an opiate medication that was initially designed for the treatment of severe chronic pain just like OxyContin. Fentanyl patches are still available with a doctor's prescription, typically in the form of an adhesive patch. Prescription fentanyl

[2] "Prescription Opioid Epidemic: Know the Facts," AMA Alliance, https://amaalliance.org/wp-content/uploads/2019/07/Opioid-White-Paper_Final_Template.pdf.

patches are applied to the skin and gradually release fentanyl into the bloodstream over seventy-two hours. After three days, the patch is then taken off the skin and replaced with another one. While prescription fentanyl patches inadvertently caused many patients to develop addiction, the fentanyl that you've been hearing about is somewhat different. The fentanyl that is killing Americans at an unfathomable rate is being smuggled into our country, typically in the form of a powder. It is now recognized that Mexican cartels are sneaking it across our southern border at an incredible rate. This fentanyl is then compressed into fake pills and sold on the street by drug dealers. Ingesting just one tiny granule of fentanyl powder is enough to kill someone in just a matter of moments. Two pounds of fentanyl is enough to kill a hundred thousand human beings. In 2023 alone, approximately twenty-seven thousand pounds of fentanyl was caught coming across our southern border. In the upcoming chapter, we'll delve deeper into the topic of fentanyl.

The question that immediately comes to mind is, why would drug dealers want to mix fentanyl into pills and risk killing their customers? The answer is two-fold. The first and more obvious reason is that with heroin, there are many hours between the wearing off of the drug and when the intense withdrawal begins. This means that someone using heroin might be able to function relatively normally for a few hours between doses; however, with fentanyl, this isn't the case. With fentanyl, people need to use it every few hours. That puts them out on the street far more frequently. This means that the drug is still profitable for dealers even if a lot of clients die, because clients use much more of it overall. There is no safe amount of fentanyl, and unlike heroin, there are no long-term users. The second, and I believe bigger, reason that a person with opioid addiction would continue to seek out fentanyl is the following: when a person is in the throes of opiate addiction, the primary goal of their life each day is just to find more drugs. Remember that opiates hijack the circuitry in the brain, which causes the addict to seek out drugs every day at the expense of everyone and everything else. Additionally, the addicted brain will intentionally seek out fentanyl over other opiates. If you were to ask most opiate addicts why they wanted to specifically use fentanyl, they would tell you it's because they hope it will make them feel even more euphoric than oxycodone or heroin. Yes, they're aware that the fentanyl can kill them, but remember that the limbic system of their brain has been hijacked by opiates, and this overpowers any rational thought processes. Drug dealers understand this very well, and so they will intentionally promote that they have mixed fentanyl into the pills they're selling.

Over the past couple of years, there have been many non-profit organizations that have started handing out fentanyl test strips to opiate addicts. The hope was that an addict would be able to quickly test their drugs to see if they contained fentanyl—and then, if an addict saw fentanyl in their drugs, they wouldn't take it due to their risk of overdosing. Unfortunately, what this experiment showed was that while addicts were actually using these testing strips, they still took the drugs—even if fentanyl was present. Why would they do that? Remember, their brain circuitry has been hijacked.

Today, drug dealers frequently add fentanyl to many other drugs including heroin, cocaine, and oxycodone pills. The fentanyl is often "pressed" with these other drugs into a pill or powder form to sell on the street. It is nearly impossible to tell which pills have fentanyl mixed into them as drug dealers put the same engravings found on the true prescription pills. At this point, nearly all pills sold by drug dealers contain fentanyl. So, if someone, even without addiction, were to try just one pill, the risk of overdose and death is significant. Consider how many people you know who have experimented with cocaine or pills at some point. Now, every instance of use carries a high risk of death. For parents raising teenagers, this fear can feel constantly overwhelming.

Should Anyone Take Opioids?

While some post-surgical pain can be controlled with over-the-counter anti-inflammatories, such as ibuprofen, many surgeries do require three to five days of opiate pain medicine. Other situations that require opiate pain medicines include chronic neurological diseases and those suffering from terminal cancer.

Those who are prescribed opiate pain medicine to help combat post-operative pain should be switched onto non-opiate medicines, such as anti-inflammatories or acetaminophen, within just a few days. By limiting our exposure to opiate drugs—both the dose and duration—we can significantly reduce the chance of developing addiction.

Think of Opioids as the Prescription of Last Resort

Knowing what we know now, I urge medical doctors and patients to view opioids as a *prescription of last resort*. Doctors now have a plethora of non-opiate medications to help control pain, such as:

- Toradol injections
- Trigger point injections (injections into the muscles)
- Epidural steroid epidural injections (to reduce nerve pain)
- Spinal facet blocks (injections into the joints between the vertebrae)
- Lidocaine injections (into muscles or around nerves)
- Lidocaine patches
- Steroid joint injections (injections of steroids into joints such as the shoulder, knee, or hip)
- NSAIDs (non-steroidal anti-inflammatory drugs)
- Muscle relaxers
- SNRIs (serotonin-norepinephrine reuptake inhibitors), such as Cymbalta or Effexor
- Oral steroids, such as prednisone
- Gabapentin
- Acetaminophen
- Medical marijuana (more on this later)
- Non-pharmacologic modalities including chiropractic and acupuncture

Because we're not yet able to determine who is genetically susceptible to developing addiction, it is critical that you or your loved ones avoid taking any opiate pain medications unless it's absolutely necessary. Even in those instances, opiate pain medications should only be taken in the lowest amounts possible and for the shortest periods of time. It's also critical to remember that someone who is in recovery from opiate addiction, even if they have been completely sober for many years, should never take even a single dose of the drug. I have witnessed thousands of people, with many years of sobriety, fall back into full-blown addiction after just a one-week prescription from their dentist.

FENTANYL'S GRIP ON AMERICA

I n recent years, the United States has been grappling with a devastating opioid crisis, with fentanyl emerging as a particularly lethal component. Fentanyl exacts a devastating toll, claiming the lives of one hundred thousand Americans annually. Behind the statistics and headlines lies the human toll of the fentanyl crisis. Families are torn apart, communities are ravaged, and lives are lost prematurely.

Similar to many opioids, fentanyl was originally developed to manage intense pain, such as that resulting from cancer or immediate post-surgical recovery. Fentanyl is different than other opioids like oxycodone, hydrocodone, or heroin because of its potency. Its potency far exceeds that of other opioids, making even the smallest doses potentially lethal. It is estimated to be fifty to one hundred times more potent than morphine. This heightened potency increases the risk of overdose, as even small amounts of fentanyl can lead to respiratory depression and death.

Fentanyl has now flooded the streets of America, typically being added to other drugs such as heroin, cocaine, and counterfeit prescription pills, oftentimes without the knowledge of the user. Fentanyl's potency means that users may inadvertently ingest a fatal dose when consuming substances that have been contaminated with even small amounts of the drug. Fentanyl has completely transformed the landscape of drug addiction and overdoses unlike any other substance in history. Previously, it was widely recognized that maintaining an addiction to opioids like heroin or consuming high doses of oxycodone pills greatly increased the risk of fatal overdose. However, with fentanyl, the danger has escalated to a point where virtually anyone is vulnerable. It's no longer just about individuals succumbing to addiction; now even teenagers as young as sixteen, merely experimenting with drugs at a social gathering, are at risk of sudden death. Parents, take heed: even if your child isn't grappling with addiction, a single instance of drug experimentation can prove fatal. This heightened risk isn't solely attributable to fentanyl's potency; it's also a consequence of the pervasive practice of lacing fake pills, marijuana, cocaine, and other substances with minuscule amounts of fentanyl, leading to lethal outcomes from just one exposure.

While many know that fentanyl's precursors come from China, what's less recognized is China's extensive involvement at every stage of the chain that leads to American fatalities.

These precursors arrive at the port of Manzanillo in Mexico, operated by a Chinese company. From there, they are transported to a Mexican border town where two thousand Chinese nationals assist in the conversion process to fentanyl, using pill presses sourced from China and supplied to drug cartels at minimal cost.

The manufactured pills enter the United States through the border. Mexican cartels ensure secure communication using Chinese apps and devices, trusting that China will not disclose information to US authorities.

Furthermore, the laundered profits from fentanyl sales, once destined for Latin American banks, now find their way into Chinese banks.

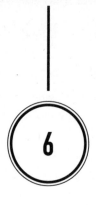

BREAKTHROUGH SCIENCE: A TALE OF TWO BRAINS

Addiction is the most widely misunderstood medical condition in all of health care, not only by the public but also by the so-called experts. Just like a person with cancer would seek the help of a cancer specialist called an oncologist, someone with addiction must seek out a physician who is board-certified in addiction medicine. This seems intuitively obvious, but what if I were to tell you that this is almost never the case? Even for those who are suffering from the agonizing and unrelenting hell of opiate addiction, less than 1 percent will ever have the opportunity to be prescribed lifesaving medication. What you are about to learn in the next few pages will fundamentally change your understanding of the brain and what happens to it with addiction. Please turn off all distractions, quiet the outside noise, and give 100 percent of your focus to what you are about to read.

Addiction is essentially a tale of two brain centers: our conscious/thinking brain (cortex) and our unconscious/automatic brain (limbic system). As you can see from the image below, the thinking part of our brain is called the cortex, and it is located in the frontal region. The automatic part of our brain is the limbic system, and it's located near the brain stem.

Let's discuss the brain's limbic system first:

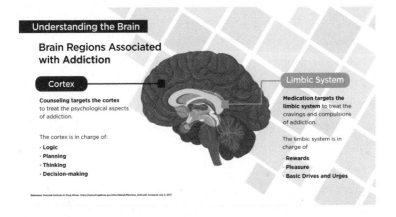

Very deep inside the brain, we have a critical center known as the limbic system. This is the command center that controls all of our basic survival drives such as eating, drinking, and procreating, as mentioned earlier in chapter 3. This part of our brain is the most powerful driver of our behavior and yet it operates completely separate from our conscious control! It's absolutely critical for you to remember that we do not have any control over this part of our brain. The limbic system not only controls our survival drives but also is in charge of running our entire autonomic nervous system. The autonomic nervous system runs all of our organs and cells, every moment of every day. The limbic system has millions of wires (neurons) that connect to the cortex part of our brain, so that when it needs to send signals to the "thinking" part of our brain, it can do so rapidly and with tremendous power. However, as you are about to learn, our thinking brain does not have the wiring that allows it to control our limbic system. This is by miraculous design! Have you ever tried to use your thinking brain to forget about your hunger? How long were you successful? It is essentially impossible because nature designed the unconscious limbic system to be far more powerful over our drives than our conscious, cortical system—this ensures our survival.

On the other hand, it's the frontal cortex that is the conscious, thinking part of our brain. Remember, this is the part of the brain that responds to situations with good judgment and an awareness of long-term consequences. Understanding the dynamic between the two different regions of our brain (the cortex/conscious versus the limbic system/unconscious) is key to understanding how drugs cause addiction. Repeated exposure to addictive substances such as opiates or alcohol disrupts the wiring of our limbic system, hijacking its normal function. This crucial brain center then perceives the drug as essential for survival, surpassing even the need for food and water. Consequently, the limbic system becomes reprogrammed, driving the individual to compulsively seek and use the drug, even with its detrimental effects.

Each person struggling with the consequences of opioid addiction realizes that the drug is the main reason for their suffering. They can see and understand this logically. However, their brain's limbic center keeps sending strong signals, urging them to continue using the drug despite the devastating harm they're causing. And remember, no matter how well-intentioned a person may be, the rational brain does not even have the wiring to send signals back to the limbic system to stop it! Every morning, the rational mind of an opiate addict grapples with the wreckage caused by the drug and yearns for cessation. However, the overpowering limbic system intervenes, enticing with promises of just one more dose. In this relentless tug-of-war, the formidable limbic system continues to win that battle. This cycle persists each day until the individual receives life-saving medication or has an overdose and dies.

But how do drugs like opiates or alcohol actually hijack the brain? To truly understand how the hacking of the limbic system occurs, you must first understand what happens when you engage in a naturally pleasurable activity. When you enjoy a tasty meal, like your favorite pizza or a delicious dessert, your body releases chemicals called endorphins. These endorphins act like natural painkillers and make you feel good. They attach to special receptors in your brain called opiate receptors. This connection causes another chemical called dopamine to be released. This dopamine makes us feel good and at the same time "teaches" our limbic system that those activities should be repeated on a daily basis. The limbic system of the brain "sees" the amount of dopamine that is released by a specific behavior and then uses it to understand which activities it must make us repeat each day. This is a concept called salience. Salience refers to the different degrees of motivation that we have toward different activities. If we didn't have such a system, and every activity felt the same, we wouldn't feel motivated to do anything in life. We would stop eating and procreating! This brain system is how nature ensures that we are motivated each day to do those things that are essential for our survival.

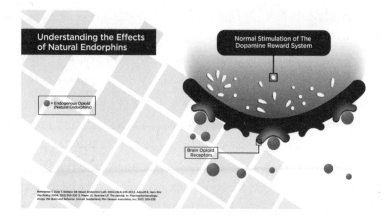

Now that you understand this key concept, let's take a look at how alcohol impacts this system. Why do most people enjoy drinking alcohol? When you drink alcohol, it raises your levels of endorphins, which then bind to those same opiate receptors, releasing a large amount of dopamine into the limbic system. This makes most people feel good and become more sociable after having an alcoholic drink. For the vast majority of people, who are not genetically susceptible to alcohol addiction, alcohol does not spike dopamine to a level that is capable of hijacking the limbic system. In other words, yes, it's enjoyable to have a drink or two, but once the evening is over, you're not going to feel compelled to drink alcohol every day. However, for some individuals who are genetically susceptible to alcohol addiction, the amount of dopamine that spikes when they have a drink is far greater. It is this enormous spike in dopamine, which happens in only about 5 percent of the population, that rewires their limbic system and then sets off compulsive cravings. Therefore, please remember the fact that what happens in one person's brain when they drink alcohol can be quite different than in another's. This is why an alcoholic, even after years of sobriety, can never safely have a single drink of alcohol—while most other people can pour a drink, have a few sips, and put it down without a second thought. The amount of dopamine gets released in the brain in response to a given drug is dictated by our genetics.

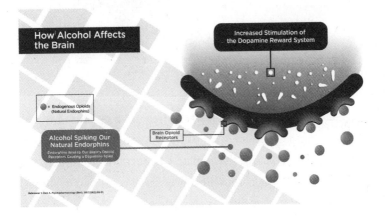

When you take an opiate drug, whether prescribed or off the street, it directly binds to the opiate receptors and causes an utter explosion of dopamine into the limbic system, one that is five to ten times greater than any naturally occurring reward in life. The limbic system, engulfed with this dopamine, will then drive the rational brain of that individual to obsessively look for opiates at the expense of everything else. This is why individuals struggling with opiate addiction often appear emaciated; their desire for food diminishes as their urge to seek and consume the drug takes precedence. It's also the reason why many individuals with opioid addiction resort to criminal activities, frequent incarcerations, and even prostitution, all in pursuit of obtaining the drug for "just one more day."

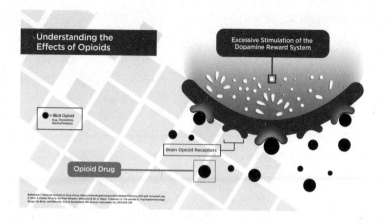

In summary, any drug addiction (regardless of the drug) is caused via this same exact brain pathway. Once the limbic system is hijacked, it then drives the addictive behavior with unrelenting force, and the thinking/conscious brain is ill-equipped to stop it. Drug use will then continue each day regardless of how much it destroys an individual's life or the life of loved ones. Free will and rational thinking alone aren't enough to stop the vicious cycle of addiction.

Importantly, individuals struggling with addiction aren't condemned to a perpetual state of suffering, merely waiting to die. In the following chapter, I'll outline the potential risks and benefits associated with the opioid addiction medications, methadone and Suboxone. If you're not yet familiar with these treatments, chances are you'll encounter them soon. There are a myriad of different opinions regarding these medications, both from doctors and from the public. It's time everyone learned the truth. After that, you will learn about breakthrough, lifesaving medical treatments that are available right now!

PART II

THE EVOLUTION OF MEDICATION-ASSISTED TREATMENTS: METHADONE, SUBOXONE, AND THE RISE OF VIVITROL

METHADONE AND SUBOXONE UNMASKED

Researchers have made significant strides in recent years in our understanding of how drugs can hijack the brain and how these neurological changes can entrap individuals in a life of addiction. As a result, we now have access to advanced neurological medications that can help alleviate needless suffering and save countless lives.

Instead of providing people with medication to help treat their condition, in the US, common approaches to treating opioid addiction still include undergoing completely ineffective standalone psychosocial approaches such as equine therapy and meditation. While such programs often rely heavily on hope, mindfulness, and religion, they overlook the physiological realities of addiction, in particular, the debilitating withdrawal that occurs when regular opioid users attempt to suddenly stop. When the brain is continually exposed to opioids like heroin, fentanyl, and oxycodone, this interrupts the body's natural endorphin production. Consequently, the brain is then reliant on these external drugs for homeostasis. Abruptly stopping opioids causes the brain to release intense stress signals, leading to opioid withdrawal—a brutal physiological process. In any other medical field, favoring prayer alone over proven medication would be considered malpractice.

A multitude of studies have now conclusively demonstrated that medication-assisted treatment (MAT) for addiction is far superior to counseling alone. In fact, drug rehabilitation programs that do not incorporate MATs continue to shut down as their success rates at helping their patients are abysmal.

These safe medications target the specific brain regions (i.e., limbic system) that have been altered by drug addiction. These MATs dramatically reduce relapses, greatly improve chances of survival, and can positively change the trajectory of one's life. In fact, the prestigious medical journal *The Lancet* refers to MAT as the gold standard for addiction treatment.

At present, there are three medications approved by the FDA to treat opioid use disorder: methadone, buprenorphine (commonly known by its brand name Suboxone), and Vivitrol. Similar to how opioids such as Percocet (oxycodone), Vicodin (hydrocodone), heroin, and fentanyl are widely recognized by name, many individuals are now becoming familiar with the medications being used to treat addiction.

The overdose epidemic has burned through the US for nearly thirty years. For much of that time, the only two medications highly effective at preventing overdose deaths were methadone and Suboxone, as Vivitrol came later. Methadone and Suboxone, both opiate-based drugs, work by replacing the opiate drug that the individual is addicted to. While many are quick to judge this as simply "switching" one opiate for another, this is not the case. This is because methadone and Suboxone are structured differently from the opiate drugs people commonly get addicted to, like oxycodone and heroin. The evidence for efficacy is overwhelming. According to NIDA, patients on methadone and Suboxone are 59 percent and 38 percent less likely to die of an opioid overdose compared to those not receiving these medications. Another study showed that incarcerated people taking methadone or Suboxone were less likely to die of an overdose in the first month after being released. This is why the World Health Organization lists both of these drugs as essential medications.

A prescription for Suboxone or methadone means someone suffering from addiction no longer has to meet with drug dealers, expose themselves to hepatitis and HIV from injecting drugs with dirty needles, risk using a lethal amount of fentanyl, or continue a downward spiral on the path of criminality, which is often necessary to pay for their drugs. Receiving a prescription for Suboxone or methadone from a physician in a regulated environment allows an individual the ability to get their life back on track. These medications are typically taken once or twice a day and satiate drug cravings, thereby preventing relapses.

Yet, while these medications are proven to help save lives, it is important to remember that they are still opiate drugs. This means that if an individual were to stop taking their medication for even one day, they would experience the same drug withdrawal they had when they discontinued using other opiates like oxycodone or heroin. This does not necessarily mean that one must stay on Suboxone or methadone for the rest of their life. These medicines can be gradually tapered off once an individual has shown that they have changed their life sufficiently such that they won't immediately relapse once the medicine has been stopped. Most human beings have an inherent bias about using ongoing medication to treat addiction and help prevent relapse. It's based on the inaccurate feeling that addiction is rooted in a psychological/behavioral problem and that people "don't need medicine." You must remember, though, that the drug addiction has chemically hijacked critical circuitry in the brain. Never forget that addiction is a deadly neurological illness! This is why there are many people who need to stay on Suboxone or methadone, for most of their life, not unlike ongoing medication for hypertension or diabetes. It can mean the difference between life and death.

For simplicity purposes, I have described methadone and Suboxone as one category. Now let me explain the subtle differences between the two.

Methadone

Methadone has been used for the treatment of opiate addiction since 1964. It is an opiate-based drug available in liquid, powder, and tablet form that is taken once a day. The only way to get methadone is to actually go into a methadone clinic. A private physician, regardless of their specialty, by law cannot prescribe methadone for the treatment of addiction. In order to receive methadone at a methadone clinic, you must regularly meet with the clinic doctor and undergo urine drug testing. The prescription is dispensed to the patient at the clinic itself—it is not sent to any pharmacy. When a person initially enters treatment into a methadone clinic, they will typically have to travel to the clinic on a daily basis to get a single daily dose. As their sobriety time lengthens, so does the amount of "take home" methadone that the patient is given.

Methadone works as a means of "replacement therapy." This means that it binds to opiate receptors in the brain, thus satiating the hijacked limbic system. This stops the individual from going into withdrawal and shuts down compulsive behavior and unrelenting cravings.

One of the problems with methadone is that it is a "full opioid agonist." This is a medical term that means that the higher the dose of methadone taken, the more and more it will impact the brain—without any ceiling on that effect. What does that mean? It means that if someone were to take more methadone than prescribed, then they could start to feel "high" or euphoric just like the opiate drugs that they were abusing in the past. This also means that if someone were to take enough methadone, they could overdose and die.

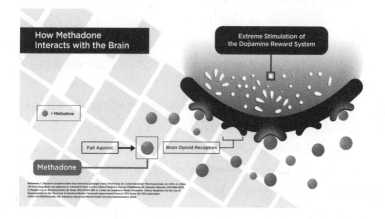

Buprenorphine (Suboxone)

Buprenorphine was approved by the FDA for the treatment of opioid addiction in 2002. Buprenorphine is the active ingredient in the medicine Suboxone. (Suboxone is the brand name.) For simplicity's sake, throughout this book I will use the term Suboxone rather than buprenorphine. In my view, Suboxone is far superior and safer than methadone.

Like methadone, Suboxone is also opiate-based and is considered a "replacement therapy." Suboxone, however, can be prescribed by a physician in a private office. This means that there is typically more privacy and less hassle, as compared to traveling to a methadone clinic. Additionally, Suboxone is a "partial agonist," as compared to methadone, which is a "full agonist." What this means, essentially, is that beyond a certain dosage, Suboxone can no longer stimulate the brain. Consequently, even if you were to take double or triple the prescribed dosage of Suboxone, it would not cause you to have a drug overdose. This "partial agonist" mechanism also means that there is less potential for people to feel high. The vast majority of people who are stable on Suboxone will tell you, "I just feel normal, and I don't have any cravings for drugs."

Remember, just like methadone, Suboxone is also an opiate-based medication. This means that if you were to suddenly stop taking Suboxone, you would experience the same withdrawal symptoms as coming off methadone or any other opioid drug. Remember that regardless of whether it's methadone or Suboxone, tapering off these medicines should be directed by a physician so that it's done safely.

Unlike with methadone, you do not have to visit a specialized clinic in order to get the medication. Suboxone is typically prescribed by a physician in a private office–type setting, as mentioned earlier, and the prescription is filled at a local pharmacy. The doctor determines how long the prescription is written for, and it can range from one day to one month at a time, based on how well the patient is doing with their recovery. Suboxone is typically taken as a sublingual (under the tongue) or buccal film (placed against the inside of the cheek) once per day. (There is some variation to the frequency, as some patients may be prescribed the medicine twice or even three times per day.)

In 2017, Sublocade—a once-monthly injection of buprenorphine (the active ingredient in Suboxone)—was approved by the FDA. If the decision is made to treat a patient with Suboxone, opting for this once-monthly injection offers several advantages over prescribing daily Suboxone films. The Sublocade injection mitigates various risks associated with Suboxone, such as the possibility that a patient may not adhere to their daily dosage regimen. Some patients might intermittently take their prescribed Suboxone but permit themselves "a day off" and use street drugs like heroin or fentanyl on the so-called day off to get high. Additionally, because of its opioid-like properties, some people experience an increased sense of well-being. Consequently, it commands a street value, prompting some individuals to sell their prescribed doses.

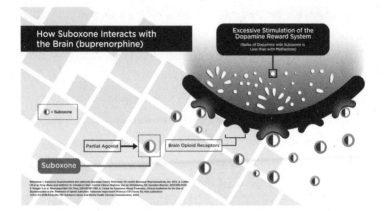

It's critical to remember that both methadone and Suboxone save lives. Overwhelming research backs this conclusion. If you or someone you love is stuck in opiate addiction, either of these medications is a better option than what will inevitably happen from continually buying and using drugs from a drug dealer. Despite the overwhelming evidence showing how critical these medicines can be for survival, there is still a tremendous stigma. When it comes to addiction, maintaining a stigma against these medicines is extraordinarily dangerous as it can prevent people from getting the medicine they need to stay alive.

While methadone and Suboxone are the most widely known medications to treat opiate addiction, they are not the only medically prescribed treatments available. Keep reading, because you are about to learn incredible information about a new, non-habit-forming prescription medicine that treats both opiate and alcohol addiction, called Vivitrol!

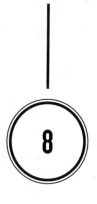

VIVITROL: REVOLUTIONIZING ADDICTION TREATMENT

In fighting the opioid crisis, the names Suboxone and methadone have become household words. This is not at all surprising as 95 percent of doctors choose these medicines as their first-line prescriptions for the treatment of opioid addiction. But did you know that there is a third lifesaving medical treatment that far fewer know about? It's a miraculous medicine called Vivitrol, and it's a once-monthly injection that's FDA-approved for the treatment of both opiate and alcohol addiction. (While the focus in this chapter will be the utilization of Vivitrol for opioid addiction, later in the book I will further describe its role in the treatment of alcohol addiction.)

What Makes Vivitrol Different?

Vivitrol is the newest medical treatment for combatting opiate addiction, and it stands in stark contrast to Suboxone or methadone. Vivitrol, unlike Suboxone or methadone, is not an opioid-based medication and is therefore not habit-forming. This means that a person who is treated with Vivitrol experiences recovery in a more "sober" state than those who are on the other two drugs. Additionally, if and when the determination is made for medication-assisted treatment to stop, those on Vivitrol can simply stop without experiencing any withdrawal symptoms. This is most definitely not the case with Suboxone or methadone, because with these medicines, one must be tapered very slowly over several months or years in order to avoid terrible withdrawal symptoms.

There is, however, a far greater reason to choose Vivitrol treatment over those other forms of MAT. When a person is on Suboxone or methadone, the brain doesn't have a chance to return back to its more normal number of opiate receptors. Additionally, the emotional centers of the brain, like the amygdala, aren't allowed to reset to lower thresholds, and the hippocampus continues to lay down memories in the presence of an opioid-based drug.

Although this has not yet been proven, it is my opinion as a neurologist and addiction specialist that Vivitrol is actually helping to "heal" the brain. While we don't know if it's possible to fully revert the brain back to the state it was in prior to the addiction starting, I believe Vivitrol offers the closest path possible.

Vivitrol is a once-monthly intramuscular injection that can be given in a private doctor's office. The active medicine in Vivitrol, known as naltrexone, is gradually released from the muscle and into the brain over the following twenty-eight days. Within just a few hours of receiving their first Vivitrol injection, many people report a dramatic reduction in their cravings or desire to use opioids. On page **76**, you will find a chart highlighting the key differences between methadone, Suboxone, and Vivitrol.

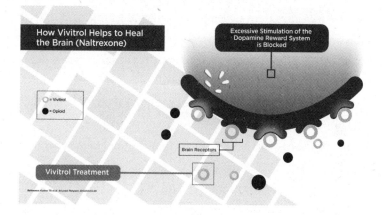

There was much excitement when Vivitrol won FDA approval in 2010 for the treatment of opiate-use disorder. Finally, there was a powerful, safe, and non-habit-forming medicine that could transform the lives of those who seemed helplessly addicted. We are now fourteen years since its release and still less than 5 percent of doctors are offering it to their patients as a first-line treatment for opioid addiction. What happened?

There are a number of reasons why you've probably never heard of Vivitrol. I believe that one of the biggest reasons is that doctors rarely ever choose to prescribe it. My experience from teaching across the country is that most addiction doctors believe that it's just too challenging because of the detox process that's required prior to starting Vivitrol treatment. This may sound confusing, so I will explain it in more detail.

First, let's review the process of initiating someone with opioid addiction on Suboxone. The entire procedure is completed in just one day. Typically, the process involves instructing the patient to cease all use of the opioid drugs they are currently abusing. Once their bodies have developed significant opioid-withdrawal symptoms (typically about sixteen hours later), then they place the Suboxone film(s) under their tongue. Because Suboxone is an opiate-based drug, it enters the person's brain and within minutes stops the withdrawal symptoms. The patient is then given instructions on how to determine their total correct daily dose. A person on Suboxone must then wake up each day and take Suboxone (usually once or twice throughout the day so that they don't have any drug cravings or withdrawal symptoms).

The process of taking someone who is actively abusing illicit opioid drugs and starting them on Vivitrol is significantly different. Vivitrol is what's known as an "opioid antagonist." This means that Vivitrol enters the brain, binds to opioid receptors, and then shields them off so no other opioids can attach. However, unlike Suboxone and methadone, Vivitrol does not trigger any dopamine release. If that person were to have opioids still in their system when the first Vivitrol injection is administered, then the Vivitrol would instantly dislodge that opioid off the brain. This would cause that person to experience "precipitated opiate withdrawal." Precipitated opiate withdrawal refers to a person experiencing the sudden onset of severe opioid withdrawal. While this is not considered to be deadly, it can be highly uncomfortable, and so it's important to avoid this happening. To prevent precipitated opiate withdrawal, the doctor must ensure that the addicted individual abstains from all opioids for seven to ten days before returning for their initial Vivitrol injection. It is specifically this time period that concerns most addiction doctors. The fear is that during those seven to ten days, their patients won't be able to make it through the uncomfortable withdrawal process and could wind up picking up drugs again and never actually make it to their appointment for Vivitrol. As I will explain later in the book, I have developed a specific protocol of "comfort" medications that allows patients to go through opioid detox in their homes and with very minimal distress. This makes it easy for most patients to make it through that seven-to-ten-day period and then get their first Vivitrol injection. While detox protocols similar to mine have now been published in medical journals, there are still very few doctors who utilize them in practice. The bottom line: if doctors won't learn how to properly keep patients comfortable during the detox period, then it makes it all but impossible for them to offer Vivitrol to their patients.

You might be wondering if a patient could enter an inpatient detox center for those seven to ten days, ensuring they stay off all opioids during that time, and then receive their first Vivitrol injection before leaving. In theory, this could work. However, most detox programs immediately start patients on Suboxone upon admission. Why? Because Suboxone quickly alleviates withdrawal symptoms and drug cravings. Although doctors could use non-opioid medications to manage withdrawal and then start Vivitrol prior to discharge, they usually don't due to their limited training and the convenience of Suboxone. But starting and maintaining Suboxone treatment during the detox process prevents patients from getting Vivitrol. Typically, following discharge, the patient is referred to a private physician for ongoing maintenance Suboxone treatment. The duration of Suboxone treatment varies depending on the patient, lasting from a month to several years. While this treatment approach is a valid option, it doesn't leave room for starting a Vivitrol treatment.

Imagine you're someone grappling with a life-or-death addiction. You enroll in a drug treatment program, only to realize that the mandated protocol robs you of the chance to even contemplate starting Vivitrol. That is the current state of addiction treatment. You might also wonder, can't a patient just switch from Suboxone to Vivitrol later on? However, since Suboxone is an opioid-based medication, it would also need to be discontinued for seven to ten days prior to the first Vivitrol injection. Remember, stopping Suboxone triggers the same intensity of opioid withdrawal symptoms as any other opioids, including heroin or fentanyl. Therefore, unless doctors become comfortable prescribing a non-opioid-based protocol of medications to help patients remain comfortable during this withdrawal period, they will never be able to offer Vivitrol treatment.

In my training as a neurologist, I have become quite experienced in combining different families of medicines to help patients with a plethora of different neurological conditions. I knew that if I could solve this dilemma of helping patients stay comfortable through their withdrawal process without using Suboxone, then it would open the door for countless people to start Vivitrol treatment. By 2014, I had accomplished this mission and was finally able to set people free from the chains of opioid dependency. By utilizing a highly specific combination of neurological-based medicines, I was able to finally stop a person's opioid withdrawal during that seven-to-ten-day period without having to use Suboxone. For most patients, this detox protocol could be done in the comfort of their own homes. Then, after those seven to ten days, that patient would return to the office and be treated with their first injection of Vivitrol. After the first injection of Vivitrol, most patients report having no cravings for opioid drugs. Additionally, their loved ones could rest a little easier knowing that for the entire month after the Vivitrol injection, even if they were to take opioids, they would be blocked from entering the brain. Remember, if a person with Vivitrol in their system were to use opioids, then in almost all instances the Vivitrol shield would block the drug from entering the brain. This would dramatically reduce the chance of them becoming addicted again, as well as prevent them from having an overdose. The patient then returns monthly for subsequent Vivitrol injections. The plan is then to continue with the Vivitrol injection once a month for approximately six months to a year. This helps ensure that the brain is healing and that the person is able to significantly change their lifestyle before the Vivitrol shield is removed.

Over the past several years, I was able to initiate Vivitrol treatment in nearly every patient who needed it. Alkermes, the pharmaceutical company that manufactures Vivitrol, took notice of this success and asked me to teach other doctors around the country. For more than three years, I traveled and trained doctors across the United States on the protocols I created.

To date, I have personally treated hundreds of patients with Vivitrol, helping them find recovery from opiate and alcohol addiction. Virtually all patients tell us that they no longer have intense, uncontrollable cravings or even think about opioids. Since I started this journey, numerous medical studies have been published demonstrating the power and safety of Vivitrol.

It's important to remember that treating patients with a cookie-cutter, one-size-fits-all approach is rarely the best strategy. That is why I continue to use all available forms of medication-assisted treatment in my practice, including Suboxone. Not every person will respond the exact same way to a medication, including Vivitrol. That's why it's crucial for addiction specialists to be highly trained and experienced, and to have a comprehensive understanding of all available treatment options.

Vivitrol: Studies and Outcomes

- Below, you will find information about several studies conducted on the efficacy of Vivitrol for treating both alcohol and opioid addiction. To gain FDA approval for Vivitrol as an alcohol addiction treatment, a study was done in Russia (published in 2005). This six-month study included 417 individuals with alcohol addiction. Roughly half of them were treated with a placebo injection and the other half with a Vivitrol injection. Most notably, the study showed that those on the Vivitrol treatment were able to reduce their heavy drinking days by 92 percent compared to the placebo group.[3]

---

[3] Krupitsky, Evgeny, Edward V. Nunes, Walter Ling, et al. "Injectable extended-release naltrexone for opioid dependence: a double-blind, placebo-controlled, multicentre randomised trial." *The Lancet* 377, no. 9776 (April 2011): 1506–1513. https://pubmed.ncbi.nlm.nih.gov/21529928/.

- A second study done in Russia was published in 2011, which helped Vivitrol gain FDA approval for the treatment of opioid addiction. The study looked at 250 opiate-addicted people. Roughly half were treated with Vivitrol, and roughly half were treated with a placebo injection. The study revealed that those patients who received the real injection of Vivitrol reported dramatically fewer cravings for opiate drugs and were seventeen times less likely to relapse, as compared to the placebo.

- A twenty-four-week study, conducted and published in the United States in 2018 and funded by the National Institute of Drug Abuse (NIDA), compared Vivitrol head-to-head with Suboxone. Of 474 people with opiate addiction, 204 were treated with Vivitrol and 270 were treated with Suboxone. Patients treated with Vivitrol had at least the same level of reduction in their cravings as did those who were treated with Suboxone. Remember that Suboxone is a very potent opiate, and Vivitrol is not an opiate at all, yet it was just as powerful at reducing drug cravings.[4]

- Another head-to-head study of Vivitrol and Suboxone was conducted in Norway and published in 2017. Roughly half of the 159 people in the study were treated with Vivitrol, and the other half were treated with Suboxone. The patients in the Vivitrol group showed fewer

---

[4] Lee, MD, Dr. Joshua D., Edward V. Nunes Jr., MD, Patricia Novo, MPH, et al. "Comparative effectiveness of extended-release naltrexone versus buprenorphine-naloxone for opioid relapse prevention." *The Lancet* 391, no. 10118 (November 2017): 309–318, https://www.thelancet.com/journals/lancet/article/PIIS0140-6736(17)32812-X/fulltext.

days of relapsing and more days of sobriety as compared to those on Suboxone. The study also showed that more people on Suboxone decided to drop out of the study before it was completed than did those in the Vivitrol treatment group.[5]

Remember though—medication alone, whether it be Suboxone or Vivitrol, should always be combined with some form of addiction counseling. Counseling is essential for the patient to develop the coping and life skills needed to remain drug-free. How long each person is on medicine is highly individualized, but medicine should never be stopped until that individual has had time to learn coping skills to deal with life's stressors and has made a strong social support network that they can reach out to.

---

[5] Tanum, Lars, Kristin Klemmetsby Solli, Zill-E-Huma Latif, et al. "Effectiveness of Injectable Extended-Release Naltrexone vs Daily Buprenorphine-Naloxone for Opioid Dependence: A Randomized Clinical Noninferiority Trial." JAMA Psychiatry 74, no. 12 (December 2017): 1197–1205. doi:10.1001/jamapsychiatry.2017.3206.

SILENCING THE SAVIOR: THE FORCES BLOCKING VIVITROL'S REVELATION

I f Vivitrol is an FDA-approved, non-opioid, non-habit-forming medication that's highly effective in the treatment of opioid addiction, then you might be wondering why most people haven't heard of it.

In the last chapter, I explained that one of the reasons so few people are offered Vivitrol has to do with doctors' lack of knowledge/experience in helping patients through the seven-to-ten-day home detox process that's necessary in order to start Vivitrol. It requires far less skill to simply transfer someone off illicit opioids and onto Suboxone. There are, however, some other key reasons that most of the public has never heard about Vivitrol.

Treatment Facilities

In the United States, there are approximately 1,500 methadone clinics that are federally certified opioid treatment programs. Most of these clinics employ dozens of workers and generate their revenue through patient visits in which patients receive their dose of methadone. It's quite typical for methadone clinics to require patients to make multiple visits per week in order to get their methadone. If even a single dose is missed, a person could experience severe withdrawal symptoms. I call it the "methadone industrial complex." Most patients who enter methadone clinics wind up staying on the medicine for years, even decades. While it is possible for patients to switch from methadone to Suboxone or methadone to Vivitrol, this process is clinically challenging, and most doctors do not encourage it.

As discussed earlier, with the advent of Suboxone, people suffering from opioid addiction had another option that didn't require them to wait in line at methadone clinics several times a week. To gain certification for prescribing Suboxone from their private practices, doctors simply needed to complete an eight-hour course, with no requirement for additional training in addiction medicine. This loophole allowed many doctors, lacking formal addiction training, to exploit those struggling with addiction. Some doctors chose not to accept insurance from patients seeking addiction treatment, instead charging high out-of-pocket fees to prescribe Suboxone. Consequently, there was a surge in the number of doctors willing to treat addiction, but many lacked the expertise to offer treatments beyond Suboxone. This contributes to the neglect of Vivitrol treatment discussions, as doctors often lack the necessary expertise, having only completed an eight-hour course on Suboxone prescribing. Moreover, it's more financially advantageous to keep patients on Suboxone indefinitely than it is to treat them temporarily with Vivitrol.

Despite the science, sinister forces were at play to hide this treatment from the American public. Alkermes began advertising Vivitrol on billboards and in subway stations in 2017. Indivior, the pharmaceutical company that manufactures Suboxone, immediately attacked them, seemingly trying to block any competitors to Suboxone. One of the biggest names on this vocal bandwagon was then–US senator from California Kamala Harris, who today serves as vice president to President Joe Biden.

In November 2017, Harris launched an investigation into Alkermes' advertising practices and wrote a letter to Alkermes CEO Richard Pops essentially asking why the company was promoting an addiction medication other than Suboxone. The letter accused Alkermes of having spent millions on "an aggressive lobbying and marketing campaign to increase the use of Vivitrol instead of cheaper treatment alternatives, like methadone and buprenorphine [Suboxone]."

What Harris failed to mention in her letter or in the investigation she instigated, was that just three years earlier, in 2014, one of her biggest political donors—the law firm of Paul, Weiss, Rifkind, Wharton & Garrison LLP—served as legal advisor to Indivior, the maker of Suboxone. According to OpenSecrets.org, the law firm gave more than $250,000 to Harris's various campaign funds between 2013 and 2020.

Alkermes barked back, releasing a statement pointing out that Vivitrol is the only medication approved by the FDA to prevent relapse following opioid detoxification and that it is non-hab-it-forming.[6] Alkermes also blasted the addiction treatment system, saying its fragmented nature resulted in too many providers not offering treatment based on the patient's clinical needs, but instead providing a one-size-fits-all approach.

Additionally, the truth is that while the Suboxone films may be cheaper than the monthly Vivitrol shot, Suboxone is administered over decades—possibly a lifetime; alternately, Vivitrol is administered over approximately six to twelve months. Thus, Vivitrol is not significantly more expensive. Ultimately, both are usually covered by most commercial health insurance carriers.

In the last few years, Suboxone manufacturer Indivior and its then-CEO Shaun Thaxter have been charged with misleading state Medicaid programs about the dangers of Suboxone to children, violating the False Claims Act in its marketing, pumping sales to doctors who prescribed the drug for off-label use, and other related federal and state criminal claims, according to the US Department of Justice. Indivior will have to pay more than $600 million to federal and state authorities through 2027 and a whopping $1.4 billion to settle its marketing allegations. In October 2020, parent company Reckitt Benckiser Group agreed to settle with New York's attorney general and five other states that claimed its pharma division, later rebranded as Indivior, misled

---

[6] "Alkermes Responds to Senator's Inquiry," press release, November 6, 2017, http://media.corporate-ir.net/media_files/IROL/92/92211/ Alkermes Responds to Senator%E2%80%99s Inquiry.pdf.

doctors on the safety of Suboxone, leading to chronic over-pre-scription of the medication.[7]

Even the role of methadone has come under scrutiny in today's drug crisis, along with its maker, Mallinckrodt Pharmaceuticals. Mallinckrodt happens to also be the largest manufacturer of oxycodone and hydrocodone (Vicodin). In 2010, the US Drug Enforcement Administration referred to Mallinckrodt as "the kingpin within the prescription drug cartel." Mallinckrodt's liabilities could be as much as $5 billion. There are few afflictions that cause such widespread suffering and death as addiction to opioids. People who are dealing with this horrific illness should be offered all available effective treatment options, not just those that are "easiest for doctors to prescribe." Vivitrol is a phenomenal medicine; it's available now, and it's covered by virtually all insurance companies. Despite this, only 1 percent of physicians know what Vivitrol is, have received any education about it, or are willing to use this treatment.

Challenging the dominant financial interests of the "methadone industrial complex" and countering the influential lobbying of pharmaceutical corporations poses a significant hurdle. Nonetheless, considerable strides have already been taken. Vivitrol, an addiction treatment medication, is now included in prescription plans and covered by insurance across almost all fifty states. Furthermore, over forty states have implemented programs to provide Vivitrol to incarcerated individuals struggling with addiction in correctional facilities.

---

[7] "AG James, States Reach Settlement with Reckitt over Allegations of Improper Marketing of Suboxone," press release, October 23, 2019, https://ag.ny.gov/press-release/2019/ag-james-states-reach-settlement-reckitt-over-allegations-improper-marketing.

Most people aren't aware that typical head-to-head medication trials are funded by pharmaceutical companies. In an unusual move, the National Institute on Drug Abuse stepped in and fully funded a head-to-head study comparing Vivitrol to Suboxone. This study was deliberately designed to rigorously test Vivitrol, allowing doctors to prescribe patients the highest daily dosages of Suboxone. The results were clear: just one monthly dose of Vivitrol was as effective at reducing cravings as the highest dosage of Suboxone. It's important to recall that Vivitrol is non-opioid and non-addictive. The federal government's strategy to combat the opioid crisis would expand Vivitrol's use to inmates as they leave jail.[8] It also calls for federal inmates with SUD to be treated with Vivitrol while incarcerated.

8   Botticelli, Michael. "Why Trump's opioid plan falls short." STAT. March 20, 2018. https://www.statnews.com/2018/03/20/trump-opioid-plan/.

VIVITROL: FREQUENTLY ASKED QUESTIONS

How does Vivitrol work?

Vivitrol is an extended-release medication that is injected once per month. It is an intramuscular injection that is given into the buttock region. Vivitrol is administered by a health provider and not by the patient themselves. After the injection is given, the active ingredient (naltrexone) is then gradually released into the body over the following three to four weeks. The injection is then repeated on a monthly basis. The number of injections that are required is entirely based on the individual and is determined between them and their doctor.

Vivitrol is an "opioid antagonist," which means that it binds to the opiate receptors in the brain, thereby preventing any opioid drugs from being able to reach those receptors. Many people report having a dramatic reduction in their cravings for opioid drugs while on this treatment. Additionally, even if an individual were to relapse and use opioids such as oxycodone or heroin while Vivitrol was in their system, the Vivitrol would block the drug from entering the brain. This would prevent that person from feeling "high" and would greatly reduce the risk of an opioid overdose.

Vivitrol is also FDA-approved for the treatment of alcohol addiction. You might ponder how one medication can effectively address both opioid and alcohol addiction. As discussed earlier, alcohol addiction operates through a similar neural pathway as opioid addiction. When alcohol is consumed, it triggers the release of endorphins, which then bind to opioid receptors in the brain, causing a surge in dopamine in the limbic system. This intense dopamine surge can hijack the brain's reward system, especially for individuals with a genetic predisposition to opioid addiction. Once addiction takes hold within the limbic system, compulsions to continue drinking can become overwhelming. Based on my clinical experience and numerous studies, alcoholics treated with Vivitrol report significantly reduced cravings and improved control over their drinking. Vivitrol achieves this by reducing the brain's response to alcohol, diminishing its ability to trigger intense activity in the limbic system.

How is the Vivitrol treatment administered?

The medicine is injected into the upper outer region of the buttocks. The injection takes a few seconds and has very minimal discomfort.

How long must I be opiate-free before starting Vivitrol treatment?

It's important to note that Vivitrol does not treat opioid withdrawal symptoms. Instead, it is administered after the opioid detoxification process is completed to aid in reducing drug cravings and preventing relapse. This means that individuals seeking Vivitrol treatment must first refrain from all opioids, including Suboxone, for a period of seven to ten days. This timeframe is necessary because it takes seven to ten days for opioid withdrawal syndrome to subside. It is strongly advised not to discontinue opioid drugs independently, but rather to do so under the guidance of a healthcare professional. Remember that there are various non-opioid medications available to help alleviate symptoms and enhance comfort during this period. In some instances, opioid detoxification can be managed at home using these supportive medications prescribed by your doctor. However, in other cases, it may be necessary to undergo detoxification in a supervised environment, such as an inpatient detox facility. I have developed specific non-opioid-based protocols of neurologically based medicines that immediately and dramatically reduce opioid withdrawal symptoms. This has allowed me to successfully detox patients from the comfort of their own homes and treat them with Vivitrol in just three to four days after the last opioid use, rather than waiting seven to ten days. Unfortunately, most physicians are inexperienced with these detox protocols, so this option may not be available where you live.

How long should patients stay on Vivitrol?

Vivitrol is not—nor is it intended to be—a life sentence. Treatment length varies based on the individual but typically lasts for six months to one year. Based on my experience in treating thousands of people with addiction, a treatment course of at least one year provides the most success. The length of treatment is individualized for each patient to ensure that the psychological and behavioral aspects of the disease have been adequately addressed and the individual has developed the life skills needed to remain drug-free before stopping Vivitrol treatment.

It's crucial to understand that with Vivitrol treatment and sustained sobriety, an individual's tolerance to opioid drugs decreases significantly. While this isn't a concern while under the protection of Vivitrol treatment, it becomes important to remember once the treatment is discontinued. Without the protective effects of Vivitrol, the risk of overdose upon resuming opioid use becomes similar to what it was when the individual first started using drugs. This principle applies to anyone who achieves prolonged sobriety from opioids, whether with or without the assistance of Vivitrol. During the period of abstinence, the brain loses the tolerance it developed during drug use. If you were to discontinue Vivitrol treatment and resume using opioid drugs, you might be at an elevated risk of overdose. This is a common occurrence among individuals who have achieved long-term sobriety while incarcerated, only to experience immediate relapse and overdose upon release. Consequently, I strongly advocate for individuals with opioid addiction who are exiting prison to receive a Vivitrol injection before their release and be given a referral to a physician who can continue with ongoing Vivitrol treatment. This recommendation is reinforced by the fact that over forty states now offer Vivitrol treatment to prisoners.

What happens if someone takes an opiate while on Vivitrol?

Vivitrol dramatically reduces cravings, but it also acts as a blocker, putting a protective "shield" around the brain. Under typical circumstances, if a person on Vivitrol takes an opioid, that drug will be unable to bind with the brain receptors. The person would not feel high or get sick. Instead, the opiate would simply be metabolized and secreted from the body. Since Vivitrol blocks opioids, it prevents the abnormal rush of dopamine in the brain that causes the euphoric feeling of being "high" and reduces the risk of an overdose.

Although insurance typically covers Vivitrol as a monthly injection, it's essential to understand that naltrexone, the active ingredient in Vivitrol, can be metabolized at varying rates among individuals. Based on my clinical observations, approximately 10 percent of patients may experience heightened drug cravings a few days before their next scheduled Vivitrol injection. This phenomenon is particularly common during the initial months of treatment as the brain undergoes healing.

Therefore, it's crucial for patients to receive their Vivitrol injection every three to four weeks, rather than waiting the full twenty-eight days, to maintain a consistent level of the medication in the brain. However, achieving this frequency may present challenges due to insurance coverage limitations as they often will only cover the Vivitrol injection every twenty-eight days. In my practice, I have often successfully discussed this issue with insurance carriers to secure approval for Vivitrol injections every three weeks for certain individuals. In other cases, I prescribe 50 mg oral naltrexone pills to be taken daily during the week leading up to the next Vivitrol injection. This helps elevate the level of naltrexone in the brain, thereby reducing cravings while awaiting the subsequent Vivitrol injection.

Does someone need to be alcohol-free when starting Vivitrol treatment?

Unlike with opioid drugs, a person does not need to stop drinking alcohol before receiving their first Vivitrol treatment. Vivitrol will *not* induce withdrawal from alcohol in the same way that it will to a person who has opioids in their system. A person can even be treated on the same day as their last drink.

It's crucial to understand that Vivitrol is not intended for the treatment of alcohol withdrawal, just as it's not designed for opioid withdrawal. Instead, its purpose is to help alleviate cravings for the drug and prevent relapse. Therefore, individuals struggling with alcohol addiction cannot simply seek Vivitrol treatment from their doctor and expect to stop drinking without experiencing potentially dangerous withdrawal symptoms. Alcohol withdrawal can be extremely hazardous, even fatal, unless managed under the supervision of a physician. Withdrawal symptoms require management with a distinct set of medications, such as Librium, diazepam, clonazepam, or gabapentin. These medications can be initiated concurrently with Vivitrol treatment. Depending on the severity of the case, alcohol detox may be conducted at home using prescription medications or in a monitored setting such as a hospital.

In essence, while alcohol withdrawal treatment addresses the patient's symptoms, Vivitrol works to reduce cravings and sustain abstinence. As mentioned above, there is no required time of waiting between the last alcoholic drink and Vivitrol treatment. In fact, you can be started on Vivitrol the same day that you drank alcohol. This is because Vivitrol would not precipitate alcohol withdrawal in the way that it does when used for the treatment of opiate addiction. Vivitrol is typically administered on a monthly basis, the same as it is for opiate addiction, for a duration determined by both the doctor and the patient.

Studies have demonstrated that individuals who are on Vivitrol not only exhibit a reduced desire to drink alcohol but are also much more likely to consume alcohol in smaller quantities if they do drink. Numerous patients have reported statements such as, "While I'm on Vivitrol, a drink containing alcohol seems just like seltzer water to me."

Is oral naltrexone the same as Vivitrol?

A common question that I often get from patients and fellow physicians is, why can't we just prescribe oral naltrexone pills instead of using Vivitrol injections? As you've already learned, the active ingredient in the Vivitrol injection is called naltrexone. Naltrexone is a generic drug that can be prescribed in tablet form.

There are several reasons why we don't see the same degree of positive results when using oral naltrexone tablets instead of

Vivitrol injections. The primary reason, however, is the fact that the oral naltrexone tablet must be taken one to two times per day, every single day, in order for it to be effective. It's not hard to imagine the risks involved in asking a newly sober individual to make sure that they take this tablet every single day. For example, if a person were to decide not to take this tablet on any given day, and then go out and use opioids, they would have absolutely no protection from an overdose. Would you choose this option for a loved one? Compare this to an injection that only needs to be given every three to four weeks!

Is Vivitrol a new medication?

Vivitrol was granted FDA approval in 2006 for treating alcohol use disorder and in 2010 for opiate use disorder.

How much does Vivitrol cost?

Vivitrol is included in Medicaid coverage and is accepted by almost all private health insurance plans. Without insurance, the cost of Vivitrol is around $1,300. However, it's important to note that Alkermes offers discount cards for uninsured individuals, which substantially lower the price.

Who can administer Vivitrol injections?

Any doctor can administer a Vivitrol injection without needing specialized certification. However, it's important to note that fewer than 0.1 percent of doctors specialize in addiction medicine, and those who do not may often feel uncomfortable providing this treatment. Even physicians who have taken the eight-hour course to prescribe Suboxone may lack the advanced training required to utilize Vivitrol effectively. One of the most effective ways to find a doctor offering Vivitrol treatment is by visiting Vivitrol.com for a list of providers in your area.

What is the difference between Suboxone or methadone and Vivitrol?

Methadone and Suboxone are both "opiate-based drugs" that are used for the treatment of opioid addiction. They can typically be started within just one day of the last illicit opioid use. These medications bind to opioid receptors in the brain and quickly stop opioid withdrawal symptoms as well as drug cravings. In most situations they are continued for months or years in order to better protect the person from relapsing. Because both methadone and Suboxone are opioid-based drugs, you can't suddenly stop using them due to severe opiate withdrawal symptoms. One difference between methadone and Suboxone is the fact that methadone must be obtained from a methadone clinic that you usually must visit several times per week. Suboxone, on the other hand, can be prescribed in a private doctor's office and typically requires less frequent visits to get the medicine. Vivitrol stands in stark contrast to methadone and Suboxone due to its distinct characteristics. Unlike methadone and Suboxone, Vivitrol is not opioid-based, isn't classified as a controlled substance, and doesn't lead to dependency. It's administered as a once-monthly injection and can be discontinued without triggering withdrawal symptoms.

However, it's essential to understand that Vivitrol doesn't alleviate opioid withdrawal symptoms. Thus, individuals must refrain from opioid drug use for seven to ten days before their first Vivitrol injection. This requirement can pose a challenge for many patients unless their doctor prescribes non-opioid comfort medications to manage withdrawal symptoms during this period. As mentioned earlier, I've developed protocols to expedite Vivitrol injections within just three to four days after the last opioid use while providing comfort from withdrawal symptoms. However, there are very few physicians who offer such a protocol.

MAT Comparison

	Methadone	Suboxone	Vivitrol
Potential for Abuse	YES	YES	NO
Causes Physical Dependency	YES	YES	NO
FDA Controlled Substance	YES	YES	NO
Setting	Must attend a specialized Methadone clinic	Prescribed in a physician's office	Administered in a physicians office
How to Obtain Medicine	Only at a licensed methadone clinic	Can be picked up from a local pharmacy. Sublocade injection is mailed to your physician's office monthly	Local pharmacy or mailed to the physicians office each month.
Requires Detox Prior to Starting Treatment	NO	NO	Yes (Approx. 1 week).
Form of Medicine	Tablet or Liquid	Sublingual or buccal film (typically taken once or twice/day) Once monthly injection calle "Sublocade"	Once monthly injection
Lowers Testosterone levels	YES	YES	NO
Stopping the Medicine Requires Tapering	YES	YES	NO

Can Vivitrol help with other forms of addiction?

The FDA has only approved Vivitrol for the treatment of opiate-use disorder and alcohol-use disorder. Recall that naltrexone is the active ingredient in Vivitrol. There are several studies indicating that Vivitrol injections (or even naltrexone tablets) can help with numerous different forms of addiction, including binge eating and gambling addiction. This makes sense when you understand that all addiction takes hold by hijacking the same limbic system of the brain. Vivitrol "shields" the limbic system from allowing addictive substances or behaviors to take hold in this region of the brain. A recent study showed that spraying a specific form of naltrexone into the nasal passages of people with gambling disorders gave them much better control over their excessive gambling compulsions. In addition to the treatment of opiate and alcohol addiction, I've had enormous success in my practice using Vivitrol injections to treat both binge-eating disorder and gambling addiction. Using Vivitrol to treat conditions other than opiate or alcohol addiction is considered "off-label" by the FDA. This means that insurance companies are unlikely to cover it when used for those other conditions.

I have heard of people becoming sad after their first Vivitrol shot. Does Vivitrol cause depression?

All medications that have an impact on the brain can potentially cause a range of different neurologic and/or psychiatric side effects. In the studies done with Vivitrol only a very minute percentage (single digits) reported any symptoms of depression. For comparison, most psychiatric medications, including even anti-depressants, also have some risk of causing depression. In my experience in treating thousands of patients with Vivitrol, I have never had a case in which Vivitrol actually caused depression. In fact, from my experience, patients I've treated with Vivitrol maintained sobriety longer and had improved mental health overall when compared to those on Suboxone treatment.

The first Vivitrol injection is often given right after people have been weaned off opioids—at the exact time when low mood is very much expected, due to the withdrawal syndrome. It's my opinion that many clinicians may be mistaking their patients' low mood as being caused by the Vivitrol injection, when it is actually because their patients are still experiencing the aftereffects of opioid withdrawal. In fact, a study published in the *Journal of Psychiatry and Neuroscience* showed that patients on naltrexone (the active ingredient in Vivitrol) experienced an improvement in their depression symptoms. Experienced physicians are able to simultaneously treat the malaise or low-grade depression that often results from stopping opioid drugs.[9]

What is the most common side effect of the Vivitrol shot?

According to studies, headaches are the most common side effect of Vivitrol, although I rarely observed this in practice. Even when they do occur, in my experience, the headaches are relatively mild and resolve within a few days to a couple of weeks. Should you develop any negative physical or mental health symptoms

---

[9] Dean, Angela J., John B. Saunders, Rod T. Jones, et al. "Does naltrexone treatment lead to depression? Findings from a randomized controlled trial in subjects with opioid dependence." *Journal of Psychiatry and Neuroscience* 31, no. 1 (January 2006): 38–45. https://www.ncbi. nlm.nih.gov/pmc/articles/PMC1325065/#:~:text=In%20the%20 subset%20of%20subjects,with%20those%20on%20methadone%20 maintenance.

after being treated with Vivitrol it is critical that you tell your doctor immediately.

How does Vivitrol heal the damage opiates and alcohol have done to the brain?

There have never been studies to prove whether Vivitrol actually "heals" the brain from addiction. It has been my experience that those who are treated with Vivitrol experience their recovery differently than those on Suboxone or methadone. Unlike opioid-based treatments such as Suboxone or methadone, Vivitrol allows the limbic system in the brain to reset closer to its natural state.

Can I safely switch a patient from Suboxone to Vivitrol?

Yes. But remember, Suboxone is an opioid, so it has to be stopped a few days before starting Vivitrol. A doctor who knows how to use non-opioid comfort medications can help with withdrawal symptoms during this transition. Experienced addiction doctors can do this quickly and with little discomfort. The speed of the transition is unique to each individual's goals and how skilled their doctor is. This transition should never be attempted without the direct guidance of a physician.

PART III

PATHWAYS TO RECOVERY: 12-STEP SUCCESS, RELAPSE RESILIENCE, AND SUSTAINED SOBRIETY

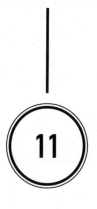

LOST IN THE MAZE: NAVIGATING THE COMPLEX WORLD OF ADDICTION TREATMENT PROGRAMS

Chances are, you've come across terms like "inpatient rehab," "outpatient rehab," and "intensive outpatient program" when it comes to addiction treatment. But figuring out what these mean and which one is right for you can be overwhelming. Adding to the confusion, some people posing as "sober counselors" might not be looking out for your best interests. In fact, they might be getting paid to send you to certain rehab centers without telling you. This chapter aims to help you understand these treatment options and avoid potential pitfalls.

Understanding Treatment Options

Understanding that recovery paths vary for individuals, for nearly everyone grappling with opioid addiction, the initial step must involve detoxification. Withdrawal from opioids is excruciating; it includes intense shaking, profuse sweating, gastrointestinal distress, agonizing restless legs, severe insomnia, and even suicidal thoughts. Attempting detoxification independently at home is typically unsafe and ineffective. Instead, detox should occur in a specialized facility or hospital. It's critical to recognize, however, that detox solely addresses the physiological withdrawal from the drug—it's not a treatment for addiction itself. While detox is a crucial starting point, it's just that: a beginning. It's akin to opening a door, but the journey of recovery truly starts after detoxification is completed. Consider this analogy: if detox were the cure for addiction, sending someone solely to detox would solve their addiction. However, reality tells a different story. Often, individuals who solely undergo detox without further treatment find themselves in a cycle, repeatedly returning to detox without addressing the underlying addiction.

Transitioning to Inpatient Rehab

After detox, most people should be transferred to an inpatient rehab facility. These places have both medical experts and counselors who can help treat the addiction and any mental health conditions. Be wary of places that say they only use "holistic methods." Often this means that they don't have any doctors or medical evaluations occurring at their facility. Treatment without the use of any medical oversight or any medications is an abysmal failure. Programs that don't offer medical supervision or medication-assisted treatment have a much higher rate of relapse and drug overdoses. In fact, most states will now refuse to certify a drug treatment program unless medication-assisted treatment is offered. Inpatient rehab usually lasts three to four weeks and prepares you for the next step: intensive outpatient counseling.

Intensive Outpatient Counseling and Sober Living

Intensive outpatient programs offer counseling and support while you live at home. Some people choose to stay in a "sober home" after inpatient rehab, where they have even more structure and support. Whether you go home or to a sober home, attending intensive outpatient counseling is critical. These programs can last one to six months and typically include regular visits with a doctor, counseling, and drug testing. All of this is done within a single facility.

Continued Support and Relapse Prevention

Recovery from drug or alcohol addiction is an ongoing journey that lasts a lifetime. Life after completing an intensive outpatient program varies greatly from person to person, and there's no one-size-fits-all approach. I strongly advise individuals to continue attending support groups like AA or NA, and/or meet regularly with a private therapist. The frequency of these meetings is flexible and should be decided by the individual in collaboration with their 12-step sponsor and/or therapist. Additionally, if medication is needed to manage drug cravings or mental health symptoms, regular consultations with a doctor are crucial.

THE SCIENCE BEHIND 12-STEP PROGRAMS

There has been a tremendous debate for many years by many experts regarding the benefits of counseling versus medicine to help those with addiction. Much of this debate, while well-intentioned, has been filled with misinformation. The fact is that over 99 percent of those with either opiate or alcohol addiction require a specific combination of both medical treatment and counseling. Additionally, these different treatments must follow a specific sequence in order to have the highest chance of success.

Counseling Therapies

If you were to do a quick search of counseling therapies used to treat addiction, you could spend weeks compiling a list. Some of the more commonly used forms of therapy are cognitive behavioral therapy, dialectical behavioral therapy, hypnotherapy, biofeedback, interpersonal psychotherapy, psychoanalytic therapy, and psychodynamic counseling. It's not critical for you to learn the specific nuances and differences between all these different forms of counseling. As you will come to learn, counseling can offer tremendous benefits for the maintenance of sobriety, but it must be started *after* medical stabilization of the brain has begun. However, before we move on from the topic of counseling and onto the medication component, I want to offer you a more in-depth understanding of 12-step meetings.

12-Step Programs (Alcoholics Anonymous/Narcotics Anonymous)

I have seen people struggling with addiction find tremendous therapeutic support from 12-step self-help programs such as Alcoholics Anonymous (AA) and Narcotics Anonymous (NA). Clinical experience has shown me that 12-step meetings are a highly effective form of counseling and should be considered the gold standard. This opinion is supported by a comprehensive analysis conducted by Stanford School of Medicine researchers, published in March 2020. The study review described 12-step programs as "the most effective form of counseling for addiction, more effective than psychotherapy in achieving abstinence." The study concluded that "AA works because it is based on social interaction; members give one another emotional support as well as practical tips to refrain from drinking." Twelve-step meetings are not affiliated with any religion and welcome people of all faiths, as well as agnostics. The foundation is simple: through regular meeting attendance and sharing experiences, people can help each other achieve and maintain abstinence from the substances to which they are addicted. Twelve-step programs provide structure and support, which are critically important for people recovering from addiction.

Sponsorship is one of the most important bonds forged in a 12-step program. A sponsor is someone who has maintained sobriety for an extended time, who helps guide a new member through recovery and provides strength and hope during difficult times. A sponsor also celebrates and enjoys positive moments with someone new in recovery.

In most cases, people who were dependent on drugs have learned the behavior of "escaping" chemically from every stressor or uncomfortable feeling. If those who are addicted to drugs do not learn to live life in a healthier manner, the chance of relapse is significantly higher. Completing the 12 steps, known as "the step work," includes a tremendous amount of self-reflection and growth. Learning to avoid triggers, establishing a sober support network of friends and companions, and developing healthy coping mechanisms are critical to maintaining sobriety.

Many people get their idea of 12-step programs from television and movies that often show angry, chain-smoking people talking about—and sometimes romanticizing—their lives in addiction. The actors depicting alcoholics on the screen act miserable, detached, and broken. And yes, some people, especially those in early recovery, may act that way. But someone I know who found active recovery through AA told me this: "I never attended a meeting like the ones shown in the movies. If AA were that depressing, I'd still be drinking. Hell, going to a meeting would make me want to drink!"

I don't want any of those inaccurate or preconceived notions about AA to keep people away from what can be a phenomenal, lifesaving part of their recovery. To clear up any misconceptions about 12-step programs, let me share my understanding of the 12 steps of Narcotics Anonymous. As I shared earlier, newly recovered people aren't expected to "practice" or "work" these steps on their own. They work with an experienced sponsor, using the steps as a roadmap to direct them to a new, clean and sober life.

Step One: We admitted we were powerless over our addiction, that our lives had become unmanageable.

The word "powerless" makes people feel like they have no control over their addiction. This is not at all what this step means. Notice that the verb "admitted" is in the past tense, meaning that, yes, you do become powerless when you are using the drug but that you are not *powerless once you have sobriety and can think rationally.* In fact, in becoming sober, you are empowered—you become power-*full*—and you have a choice to continue moving toward recovery or moving toward relapse. The powerlessness the first step speaks about is what happens immediately after you pick up the drink or drug again.

Father Joseph C. Martin, a Roman Catholic priest, recovering alcoholic, and renowned speaker/educator on the issues of alcoholism and drug addiction, said the "depth and the seriousness with which you will work the rest of this program will depend directly on the depth and seriousness with which you accept this first step. This is an admission of one's condition—surrender to understand your problem. It is not just an intellectual thing. This step is about truly knowing it in your gut."

If you have even the slightest *belief* in the back burners of your mind that you can possibly use "just one more time" and that somehow this time you will keep it "under control," then there is no doubt that you will continue to live a miserable and unmanageable life, just like the first step says.

Father Martin tells the following cogent story to explain the power of a 12-step program. A person struggling with addiction climbs into a boxing ring every day of their lives with a champion and gets beat up. Yet, they continue to get back into the ring each day. Years later, the addict continues to get out of bed all black and blue, crawling along the floor, heading for the ring and thinking, "How can I *not* get beat up today?" While they're putting the boxing gloves on once again, AA leans over their shoulder and says: "Don't get in the ring. If you don't fight, you won't get beat up." In other words: "If you don't take a drink, you won't get drunk."

Step Two: We came to believe that a Power greater than ourselves could restore us to sanity.

NA and AA are spiritual, not religious, programs. Members are asked to use their own understanding of a *higher power*, providing that the higher power is loving, caring, and greater than them.

Step two comes from the acknowledgment that the disease of addiction is far more powerful than the addict alone. Most have tried hundreds and hundreds of times to stop and yet always lose the battle. They cannot do it alone. Having a connection with your higher power is a critical part of maintaining sobriety throughout life.

If you do not believe in God, then why not believe in the power of the group? A group of people is surely stronger than an individual. That can be your "higher power." A room full of people suffering from addiction working to stay clean and sober one day at a time is much more powerful than any one member trying to do it alone. Use their collective strength until you develop your own.

Step Three: We made a decision to turn our will and our lives over to the care of God as we understood Him.

I personally believe in God and believe that God acts and speaks through other people. If you do not, it's enough for you to decide to follow the suggestions of the people who came into recovery before you. Use their experience to elevate your recovery and teach you how to live a sober life.

Step three is about making the decision to say, "My way no longer works. I'm going to follow the twelve spiritual principles laid out in the steps." I once heard someone say, "The moment I surrendered to NA, the universe conspired to work with me." He told me that at that moment, his obsession to use was lifted.

Steps Four and Five: We made a searching and fearless moral inventory of ourselves. We admitted to God, to ourselves, and to another human being the exact nature of our wrongs.

You will never get rid of your past. None of us will. It is there. No amount of regret, rage, or tears can change the past. *But you can address your guilt about it.* Unresolved remorse will destroy you. Right or wrong, you list what you have done in your life. You will discover that every human being has a series of the good, the bad, and the ugly.

In steps four and five, you make a list of the things that created guilt for you. Then talk about your list with another person, like a sponsor. Think about what you did in active addiction. When you recalled painful, guilt- and shame-filled memories, you reached for a drink or a drug to numb your discomfort. Working these steps starts establishing a new pattern of behavior, an appropriate way to cope with negative memories and emotions.

Steps Six and Seven: We were entirely ready to have God remove all these defects of character. We humbly asked Him to remove our shortcomings.

Once you recognize you no longer need those character defects that "served" you in active addiction, it's not hard to ask a higher power to take away those defects. Besides, was it not your desire to use and hide your consumption of alcohol or drugs that made you choose to lie, cheat, or steal? Sober people rarely act on every impulse. But it's a process. You cannot just decide one day to stop behaving that way, and *presto*—the defect in your character is gone. You need to decide that you are not going to live that way anymore. The concept here is that when you are willing to let go of those behaviors, God will take them from you. But He is not going to rip anything out of your tightly clenched fist if you're holding onto it for dear life.

It's like this: If you want to clean all the garbage out of your house, you can't call the sanitation company and ask the workers to go through your house and throw out what you no longer need. You must do it, room by room—labeling and bagging up the garbage and stuff you no longer need. Then you must bring the bags out to the curb on garbage-collection day. Then, and only then, will the sanitation workers pick up and haul away the trash.

Steps Eight and Nine: We made a list of persons we had harmed and became willing to make amends to them all. We made direct amends to such people wherever possible, except when to do so would injure them or others.

It is especially important to only do this step under the guidance of a sponsor. You need to make your list without worrying about making any actual amends, or else you might leave certain people out. This step is about clearing your side of the street, realizing your part in situations where others were hurt or damaged in some way.

Making amends is not necessarily an apology. Sometimes making amends means changing your behavior so you don't repeat the same mistake again. Many times, this is the greatest amends you can make.

Step Ten: We continued to take personal inventory and when we were wrong promptly admitted it.

By this point you discover something important: the only way to not add new people to your list of those you've harmed is by looking at your actions and behaviors daily. Ask yourself, "Have I knowingly or unknowingly wronged or hurt anyone?" When you find that you have, you need to admit the wrong as soon as possible. That's how you keep your side of the street clean.

Step Eleven: We sought through prayer and meditation to improve our conscious contact with God as we understood Him, praying only for knowledge of His will for us and the power to carry that out.

Prayer is nothing more than communication with God. The 12 steps teach you to pray for knowledge of God and the power you need to do His will. Over time, your understanding of God and your connection with this power greater than yourself will grow and deepen. Speak to God through prayer; listen to God through meditation.

Step Twelve: Having had a spiritual awakening as the result of these steps, we tried to carry this message to addicts and to practice these principles in all our affairs.

Gratitude goes beyond the word "thanks." In 12-step programs, gratitude means carrying the message of sobriety to somebody else that needs it. The loveliest definition of gratitude I have ever heard in my life is this: "the golden tray on which I offer to others what God has given me."

As you can tell, I am a huge believer in the results of 12-step programs like AA and NA to help people build new relationships and skills required for lasting recovery. However, 12-step programs are not a substitute for the medications that are often required to help stabilize a chemically hijacked brain. First, the limbic system must be "quieted" to protect against dangerous withdrawal and ongoing drug cravings, and then counseling can be helpful. Remember the order—medication, then counseling.

INTEGRATING HOLISTIC TREATMENTS IN ADDICTION RECOVERY

I n recent years, addiction treatment centers have increasingly integrated holistic treatments into their comprehensive care plans. These treatments, combined with medical and counseling interventions, offer significant benefits for individuals in recovery. However, it's crucial to understand that holistic therapies complement rather than replace the medical aspects of addiction treatment. Successful recovery typically involves medications for safe detoxification as well as ongoing medical treatment to manage drug cravings, prevent relapse, and address underlying mental health conditions.

Studies have shown that treatment programs lacking medication-assisted treatment (MAT) have significantly higher rates of non-completion, relapse, and even fatal overdoses. Despite the growing popularity of holistic treatments, there is limited research on their effectiveness when incorporated into addiction treatment programs.

Nevertheless, some alternative treatments have shown promise in supporting recovery. These treatments include equine-assisted therapy, energy medicine, art therapy, reiki, acupuncture, yoga therapy, and meditation therapy. Furthermore, chiropractic care, typically used for treating musculoskeletal problems such as neck and back pain, has shown promising results when combined with medication and counseling in addiction treatment.

Equine-Assisted Therapy

Equine-assisted therapy (EAT) involves using horses to provide self-reflective and metaphorical experiences that promote emotional growth. Horses are highly intuitive animals, often mirroring the emotions and behaviors of those around them. This interaction can help individuals gain insight into their own emotional states and develop essential skills like emotional regulation, communication, and problem-solving.

Energy Medicine

Energy medicine encompasses a range of practices that combine Eastern healing disciplines and Western science. These include:

- **Therapeutic Tai Chi**: This practice promotes balance, flexibility, and mental focus, which can be beneficial for stress reduction and overall well-being.

- **Yogic Breathing**: Controlled breathing exercises can help manage anxiety and improve emotional regulation.
- **Acupressure**: Applying pressure to specific points on the body can relieve tension and promote relaxation.
- **Craniosacral Therapy**: This gentle hands-on technique can enhance the functioning of the central nervous system.
- **Sound Vibrational Healing**: Using sound frequencies to promote relaxation and emotional healing.

Art Therapy

Art therapy provides a creative outlet for individuals to express their emotions and experiences. This form of therapy can help uncover underlying issues, reduce stress, and enhance emotional resilience.

Reiki

Reiki, meaning "universal life energy," involves the transfer of healing energy from the practitioner to the patient. This practice promotes relaxation and healing by balancing the body's energy flow.

Acupuncture

Acupuncture, a traditional Chinese medicine practice, has been used in the United States since the 1970s to treat addiction and other ailments. Auricular acupuncture, targeting specific points in the ear, can help address issues in the kidneys, lungs, and liver—organs often affected by substance abuse.

Yoga Therapy

Yoga therapy enhances vitality, reduces stress, and induces natural feelings of pleasure and contentment. These benefits are crucial for individuals striving for sustained recovery.

Meditation Therapy

Meditation promotes relaxation, mental clarity, and an overall sense of calm and optimism. Group meditation sessions in serene environments can significantly enhance the recovery experience.

Chiropractic Care

Chiropractic is a healthcare discipline focused on diagnosing, treating, and preventing disorders of the musculoskeletal system, particularly the spine. Chiropractors use hands-on spinal manipulation and other alternative treatments, aiming to align the body's musculoskeletal structure to support natural healing processes without the use of surgery or medications. The goal is to improve mobility, alleviate pain, and promote overall health and well-being.

One of the major benefits of these holistic treatments is their ability to help patients remain in treatment programs for longer periods. Research consistently shows that individuals who finish their entire inpatient treatment program are more likely to achieve better long-term recovery results. For example, a study on chiropractic care in addiction treatment revealed that patients who received chiropractic adjustments had a perfect 100 percent completion rate in their treatment program.

The Miami Study on Chiropractic Care

In 2001, a groundbreaking study was conducted by Dr. Jay Holder and Robert Duncan, PhD, a biostatistician at the University of Miami School of Medicine. This randomized clinical trial involved ninety-eight patients at Miami's Exodus drug-treatment program and was featured in the journal *Molecular Psychiatry*. The study aimed to evaluate the impact of chiropractic care on retention rates in addiction treatment programs.

The participants were divided into three groups. The first group received the regular regimen of addiction care, the second group received sham adjustments (where patients believed they received chiropractic adjustments but did not), and the third group received actual chiropractic adjustments to correct subluxations. The results were striking:

- The group receiving regular care had a completion rate of 74 percent.
- The group receiving sham adjustments had a completion rate of 56 percent.
- The group receiving chiropractic care to correct subluxations had a completion rate of 100 percent.

The study also reported that patients who received chiropractic care made fewer visits to the nurses' station and showed significant decreases in anxiety. These findings high-light the critical role of chiropractic care in improving reten-tion rates in treatment programs, which is essential for pre-venting relapse and supporting long-term recovery.

Inspired by these findings, while serving as medical director at Bridge Back to Life—an outpatient addiction treatment pro-gram with multiple centers across New York—I partnered with New York Chiropractic College to incorporate chiropractic care into our treatment plan. The outcomes were similar to those in the Miami study, with patients staying in treatment longer and experiencing improved recovery.

In conclusion, while medical-based treatments are critical for survival and foundational in addiction recovery, integrating holistic treatments can enhance retention in treatment programs and contribute to better overall outcomes. By combining medical interventions with holistic therapies, treatment centers can offer a more comprehensive and effective path to recovery, addressing the physical, emotional, and spiritual aspects of healing.

RELAPSE: THE GREATEST TEACHER OF ALL

Addiction is a chronic condition, one often marked by recurring relapses throughout an individual's life. Think of a person suffering from type 2 diabetes. That person can work hard to modify his diet and get regular exercise. But some days can be much harder than others. Even the most disciplined person will be prone to eating the wrong foods, skipping exercise, and having high blood sugar occasionally. The cravings and compulsions that occur with addiction are exceedingly more powerful than most people could ever comprehend. Remember—it just takes one relapse with opioids to cause a drug overdose. Every single time a person succumbs to using opioids, they are quite literally playing Russian roulette with their life. I am now regularly seeing seventeen-year-old kids, without any history of addiction, die from experimenting with one single pill. While these pills may seem authentic, mimicking the appearance of legitimate oxycodone prescriptions, they are, in fact, counterfeit, containing lethal doses of fentanyl. Fentanyl has now infiltrated nearly every town in America.

Scientific evidence and years of clinical experience show that most people suffering from addiction will relapse many times, and most will require multiple treatment episodes before they're able to have sustained sobriety. Many will unfortunately die from their relapses.

Once the switch of addiction has been turned on, that individual will never have the ability to use that drug in a recreational manner. Even if that person has twenty years of sobriety away from opioids, just a single oxycodone pill will light up the limbic system in their brain in such a way that it could send them spiraling into rabid drug use. This is the same for an alcoholic: it doesn't matter how many years of sobriety they may have—one drink will inevitably send them off the rails. While this does not mean that everyone in recovery is destined to continue relapsing throughout their life, it does mean that the susceptibility is there.

As you've learned, engaging in a pleasurable activity spikes dopamine. However, there's another neurotransmitter in our brain's limbic system known as glutamate. Glutamate is responsible for recording detailed memories of the surrounding environment—people, places, and things—during the dopamine spike caused by drug use. This is a primitive survival tactic in humans and animals, and it serves as a "bookmark" so we can remember how to find the food or mate that caused the spike of dopamine.

These unconscious memories are stored deep within the limbic system, specifically within a structure known as the hippocampus. When individuals encounter environmental triggers linked to these memories, they have the ability to activate the limbic system for the duration of their lives. This is why it's absolutely critical to do everything you can to change those triggers in your environment once you gain sobriety. Encountering these old environmental cues—the people, places, and things that were part of a drug-use ritual—can provoke tremendous drug cravings, leading to relapse.

Specialized MRIs show that people in recovery from addiction have their limbic systems light up instantly when seeing images of triggers that were associated with their drug use. This reaction of the limbic system happens so quickly that the rational and conscious brain doesn't even know it's occurring. Studies show that the lighting up of the limbic system in response to environmental triggers can occur years or even decades after the last use of the drug. In essence, people who have recovered from addiction have a subconscious "super memory" surrounding the cues in their environment associated with their previous drug use. The specific people they were getting high with, the sights and smells when they used drugs, or the time of day—all such factors become part of that embedded subconscious super memory and can now serve as drug triggers for relapse. Due to the constant presence of triggers in the environment and the potentially fatal consequences of even a single drug relapse, it's clear why many addiction specialists support the idea of lifelong medication-assisted treatment.

Coming out of treatment, many recovering from addiction struggle to remain sober when they return to the same environment where they used drugs. The cues are simply too powerful. While not everyone recovering from addiction can avoid all environmental cues for the rest of their lives, it's especially critical—particularly in the early days of recovery—to keep the triggers as far away as possible.

Medication-assisted treatment (or MAT, as we discussed earlier), such as Vivitrol, is lifesaving because it keeps the environmental cues that can lead to relapse muted. In other words, even when an individual is exposed to an external trigger, Vivitrol will prevent the limbic system from lighting up. Regular counseling and/or 12-step meetings provide benefits by surrounding a person in recovery with a group of like-purposed individuals. If cravings do occur, they don't have to go it alone. They can reach out to their therapist or sponsor, and/or attend a 12-step meeting where they can reinforce their cognitive tools to diffuse what they are feeling.

Many people in recovery stay attached to a counseling program indefinitely as a support tool to help them maintain their sobriety. Many create life-long relationships with the people they meet in 12-step groups. Once someone becomes sober, they often have to stop seeing their "friends," as many of them were also drug users. This can produce significant loneliness during early recovery, and that too can trigger a relapse. Meetings can help provide the opportunity to meet new friends who are willing to do other activities besides hanging out in bars or other potentially triggering environments.

It's important to realize that a relapse does not undo all of the gains made through past recovery. It's the norm in 12-step meetings to announce your "day count"—the number of days you're sober. Regardless of how long a person has maintained their sobriety, one relapse with a pill or drink—and it's back to saying, "I'm one day sober." People often feel incredibly disheartened when they must admit to themselves and others that their day count is now back to day one. The reason for this is that people in recovery often equate this to mean that they're no better off than they were the first time they ever got sober. It's critical to recognize that this isn't true! Just because the day count has reset to day one does not mean that all of the lessons and hard work they've accomplished in the past are lost. *A relapse doesn't undo all the gains made in past treatment.* Relapse doesn't remove what you've already learned. Starting over does *not* mean that they are in the same position as one who has never been through recovery, had any sobriety, and is newly sober for a few days. For many, it's the ultimate teachable moment about needing to call your sponsor when temptation arises, when triggers show up, and when the urge to use or drink grows strong.

SUSTAINING SOBRIETY: PRACTICAL STRATEGIES FOR LONG-TERM RECOVERY

No matter how effective medication-based treatments for addiction may be, they should always be viewed as medication "assisted" treatments. A plan of counseling and/or a 12-step program must be implemented in conjunction with the medication to offer the best hope for recovery.

Detox medications to stop withdrawal and then medication-assisted treatment such as Vivitrol can help dramatically calm down the hijacked limbic system of the brain, thereby reducing drug cravings, but an individual also must do their part to retrain their conscious/thinking brain.

Here are tips based on my clinical experience that, if followed, can lead to a life of recovery:

Consult with a Physician

It's crucial for individuals struggling with addiction to undergo evaluation by a board-certified physician in addiction medicine as soon as possible. Many detox and rehabilitation centers facilitate this process by connecting patients with a doctor before their discharge. With phenomenal new medication-based treatments like Vivitrol, we can greatly increase the chance of helping people achieve and maintain sobriety. Additionally, the addiction specialist can help distinguish if any comorbid mental health conditions are present, such as anxiety, depression, bipolar disorder, ADHD, etc. These conditions can and must be medically treated, along with the SUD.

Watch Out for Triggers

Once sober, stay away from the triggers of addiction—the people, places, and things that were associated with your "active using behavior." Studies have shown that even with prolonged sobriety, exposure to these triggers can reignite the limbic system of the brain (which was once hijacked by drugs). The limbic system can then send incredibly strong cravings to the conscious brain to seek drugs. Avoiding triggers is of critical importance, especially once MAT is discontinued.

Practice Complete Abstinence

Total abstinence is essential to maintaining sobriety. Non-prescribed mind- or mood-altering substances of any kind must be avoided. My clinical experience, as well as many studies, show that *patients are far more likely to relapse if they use any mood- or mind-altering substances,* even if it is not their "drug of choice." These drugs inhibit and distort the brain's ability to accurately assess situations and make good choices.

For example, I often see patients who believe they can continue to drink alcohol because their "drug of choice" is opioids. I can tell you that there is an extremely high likelihood, once they are in an inebriated state from alcohol, that they wind up making the deadly choice to "take opioids just one more time."

Participate in a 12-Step Program

Becoming a participating member of a 12-step fellowship, such as Narcotics Anonymous or Alcoholics Anonymous, has shown to be the most successful program for maintaining sobriety. It is here that the addicted person learns—often for the first time—that they suffer from a medical illness and not a moral deficiency.

Listening to others who also suffer from addiction and are honestly sharing their experience, strength, and hope can enable new members to find a better way to live, one day at a time.

Explore Psychotherapy

The CDC has shown that childhood adverse events often correlate with the onset of addiction. Many patients with addiction have traumatic histories and need emotional healing, while others are prone to anxiety, depression, and/or mood disorders.

Along with medication, meeting with a professional therapist can help with the treatment of underlying mental health symptoms, which otherwise may have been triggering a relapse. Addressing emotions like unresolved conflicts head-on in therapy can lower the chances of relapsing in recovery. In early recovery I recommend that everyone attend 12-step meetings and a private therapist, if possible, as they each offer vastly different sets of tools.

Establish Healthy Habits

Humans are strange creatures of habit. This is especially true when it comes to overcoming addiction. To break out of our old routines, we must establish healthy ones to replace the self-harming ones.

Sleep patterns, lifestyle choices, and negative relationships are a few of the primary triggers that need to be rectified if you are to live a drug-free existence. As creatures of habit, breaking them requires serious work. To successfully overcome addiction, people must not only quit drugs, but they must also break out of old routines. That means changing the unhealthy behaviors that dominated their daily life—irregular sleep, haphazard eating, risky relationships—and developing new routines that will support a healthy, drug-free existence.

Maintain Structure

Structure is also critically important in recovery. Facing life after active addiction can seem overwhelming. Developing a structured routine provides comfort and stability. Having a plan for the day keeps you on track, makes it easier to avoid drifting back into unhealthy patterns, and helps you prove to yourself that you are making progress one day at a time.

It has been said that those who fail to plan, plan to fail. For people recovering from addiction, they need to establish new, healthy habits and routines. Once they do that, those familiar, regular, and predictable patterns can help them heal and cope with the challenges that might threaten their sobriety. Having a routine reduces the anxiety of waking up in the morning and wondering, "What do I do now?" It restores a sense of control, of taking responsibility for your life beyond simply abstaining from drug use. It helps you, step by step, develop new patterns of behavior that will become your "default setting" as you build a healthy new life.

Establishing a daily routine does not mean rigidly programming every minute of every day. The objective is to structure a schedule that minimizes idle time while still allowing for some degree of flexibility.

Cultivate a Sober Support Network

Another critical component in a recovery plan and a key part of the routine is the creation of a sober support network. The bonds that develop with other participants in 12-step meetings can provide vital support and offer lasting benefits.

Unexpected bad events can sometimes curtail someone in recovery. That is why a strong support group is important. Having others with whom to share these incidents can serve as a valuable sounding board and is an important part of maintaining a healthy recovery posture.

How to Build a Healthy Routine

Here are some tips to consider when developing a daily routine, beginning with the basics:

> *Sleep*: Many people slept erratically while they were using drugs and suffer from insomnia in recovery. Sticking to a sleep schedule—going to bed and waking at the same time each day, including weekends—can help establish better sleep patterns and more restful sleep.
>
> *Employment*: If possible, maintain a regular, or at least predictable, work schedule. Unemployment leads to "free time." We've all heard that idle hands are the devil's workshop. Many people who eventually become addicted originally tried drugs out of boredom. Work relieves boredom, increases self-esteem, provides a routine, and allows you to earn money.
>
> *Diet*: Eat at set mealtimes, and do not skip meals. Keep the refrigerator and pantry stocked with healthy foods. Avoid frequent snacking, especially on junk foods loaded with sugar.
>
> *Exercise*: Get at least thirty minutes of moderate-intensity exercise every day, preferably at the

same time each day. Creating a focus on fitness is an amazing therapeutic outlet and provides a healthy release of endorphins.

Clean and organized home environment: Do not rush to climb up on the roof to replace those loose tiles. But do set aside some time every day and week to keep your surroundings clean and orderly. Do not let dirty clothes pile up on a chair, dirty dishes languish in the sink, or dust bunnies colonize the corners. The reason treatment centers require clients to make their beds isn't because they can't afford to hire housekeepers. The simple practice of taking care of your own things reestablishes a sense of ownership and accountability that is often stripped away in addiction.

Family and Friends

Nothing is more important than spending time with people close to you who nourish your spirit, validate your self-worth, and cheer on your recovery.

Having a structured plan for these everyday activities will help restore health and fitness, reduce the likelihood of boredom and loneliness, and facilitate productivity without procrastination. However, it's important not to become overly dependent on a routine and to remain flexible as new opportunities arise and unexpected events occur.

With a daily routine established and regular participation in a support group, you have the foundation in place for a successful recovery. With your commitment to openness and honesty, you can break the cycle of repeated relapse and progress toward a new, drug-free life.

BEYOND BOUNDARIES: TRANSFORMING PERSPECTIVES, STRENGTHENING FAMILIES, AND EMBRACING TELEMEDICINE IN ADDICTION CARE

SHATTERING THE STIGMA OF ADDICTION

The stigma of addiction is perpetuated by the language we use to describe those suffering from a substance use disorder. Remember that addiction is a neurological brain condition and not a character weakness or moral failing. When the public refers to people suffering from addiction as "addicts," it has a severe negative connotation. When most people hear the word "addict," it generates a visceral response, conjuring up nefarious images of what that individual might do or have done while using drugs. Using more accurate and fair language can make an imperative difference in the way we handle this epidemic and treat people suffering from addiction.

First, the term "addict" makes no distinction between someone who is still in active addiction and someone who has sustained sobriety. Imagine if you were labeled for life by the worst thing you ever did. We are more than our mistakes and our medical conditions.

Second, thinking of people with an addiction as "addicts" can lead you to dehumanize them or treat them like second-class citizens. The term suggests that they are "morally reprehensible" and "unworthy of respect." Yet, countless people in recovery are living long, rewarding, and productive lives. Individuals in successful, active recovery are more likely to give back and help others still suffering from addiction, especially if they remain involved in a 12-step program.

In my experience, I have found that labels like "addict" and drug "abuser" damage people recovering from addiction. Those labels shame and ostracize them, both within and outside the medical community, at a time when they most need acceptance and grace. Imagine if you managed to lose ten pounds in thirty days by working hard on an improved diet and regular exercise. That would be positive, encouraging, and a cause for celebration. Now imagine that while you are out for a walk, you hear someone refer to you with a derogatory slang word for obese. Would that encourage you to keep exercising? Or would that make you feel ashamed, like you don't even want to be seen in public, making you wonder why you even try to live a healthier lifestyle? The same is true for those struggling with addiction. They need support, not more criticism.

We need to separate the illness from the person who suffers from it. We do not define other sick people by their illnesses, and we should not do it to those suffering from addiction. We do not refer to individuals with mental and physical impairments as "crazies," "cripples," and "spastics." Yet most people don't think twice before labeling someone struggling with SUD an addict, dismissively defining an individual's entire identity and humanity with a single word that has overwhelmingly negative connotations. Worse than the stigma is that the term *addict* takes away the rest of the person's identity. You wouldn't say, "My best friend, the epileptic," or "My best friend, the leukemia patient." By defining someone solely by their condition, you reduce their identity to a single challenge. This is why language matters. They are human beings first, and their challenge is just one aspect of their life.

The language we use to describe people suffering from SUD influences how we frame issues and solutions—whether an individual should be punished or treated, and whether we afford them the full measure of human dignity or condemn them to cower in guilt and shame. Removing the stigma from addiction would influence funding decisions, medical research, and insurance coverage. It would help the public understand that this is a brain illness, not a moral failing. Most importantly, it would make it easier for people to seek treatment and regain their self-esteem. Simply choosing words that support and inform rather than discourage and embarrass can go a long way toward destigmatizing addiction.

The stigma of addiction has serious repercussions for an individual's likelihood of recovery. Apprehension about social ostracism, anxiety about how they will be received by the medical community, and fear of legal consequences keep many from seeking help. Even those who recover from SUD continue to be viewed with suspicion ("Once an addict, always an addict…"), making it harder to build a healthy, addiction-free life.

Tips for Language that Supports
Rather than Stigmatizes

Words to avoid: *Addict, junkie, crackhead.* Words like these pin labels on people that define them solely by their illness.

Better: *Person struggling with addiction, person with a substance use disorder, patient* (if in treatment). These phrases are more cumbersome than a single descriptive word, but they accomplish something important by putting the person before his or her illness and destigmatizing the condition.

Words to avoid: *Substance abuse, drug abuse.* Abuse is a strongly negative word, typically associated with child abuse, sexual abuse, domestic abuse, etc. It is a word that usually connotes harming another person and conveys the need for punishment rather than treatment.

Better: *Substance use disorder, addiction.* Addiction, unlike addict, refers to the condition rather than the person—a condition that can be treated—and is not a label that stigmatizes an individual.

We must fight addiction. But to do so, we must separate the illness from the individual who suffers from it. We must erase the tinge of character flaws and immorality from addictive disorders and restore dignity and humanity to the people who struggle to overcome them. Being careful about the language we use is an important step toward that end.

In Meghan Ralston's article, "The End of the Addict," she wrote, "I may be in the fight of my life with drugs, but I am not the drugs that I take. I am a fighter, a survivor—I am never merely 'an addict.' Please do not destroy the totality of who I am by reducing me to that one word."[10]

Legislative Changes Needed

Opioid addiction is a silent epidemic that requires those with a voice to speak for those who are not being heard. By bringing this issue into the spotlight, we stand a much better chance of providing essential resources to individuals grappling with addiction and in dire need of support to overcome it. I believe the following is desperately needed:

1. *Shut down the influx.* The federal government must do everything in its power to stem the flow of heroin and fentanyl coming into this country. Almost all of these drugs in the US are grown and manufactured in other countries. They pour across our border every day. Reducing

---

[10] Ralston, Meghan. "The End of the Addict." *Drug Policy Alliance.* March 23, 2014. drugpolicy.org/blog/end-addict.

the flood of these drugs into our communities will help stem the tide and save countless lives.

2. *Mandate insurers to cover treatment.* The federal and/ or state governments must continue to make it illegal for insurance companies to require prior authorization for MAT. While some progress has been made in this area, more needs to be done. It is not uncommon to have patients overdose and die while they are waiting for lifesaving medications to be "authorized" by their insurance company.

3. *Treat opiate withdrawal.* Patients in opiate withdrawal are often turned away from hospital emergency rooms. It has been incorrectly taught to doctors and insurance companies that while alcohol withdrawal is extremely dangerous, opiate withdrawal is akin to a "bad flu" and is not "life-threatening" or dangerous. The fact of the matter is that opiate withdrawal is horrendous. If that patient leaves and seeks to self-medicate their awful symptoms by using more opioids, they can certainly die.

Withdrawal symptoms affect all major bodily systems, manifesting as severe and persistent pain, uncontrollable vomiting, diarrhea, body tremors, severe insomnia, and intense drug cravings that can last for days. For some, these symptoms lead to suicidal thoughts. It's estimated that over 90 percent of patients find withdrawal symptoms intolerable within a few days, often resulting in deadly relapses. Withdrawal is a life-or-death issue every single time, for every single person. Insurance companies must approve admission to the hospital for opioid withdrawal in the same way that they do for alcohol withdrawal. Moreover, it is imperative for emergency room physicians and hospitalists to enhance their training and protocols regarding the treatment of individuals experiencing opiate withdrawal or addiction. Often, individuals who have experienced near-fatal overdoses are revived with Narcan, brought to the emergency department, and subsequently discharged, only to overdose again on the very same day.

4. *Expand the use of sober-living homes.* Structured sober housing is of utmost importance for many individuals in recovery, especially post-discharge from inpatient rehabilitation. While some may opt to return home and engage in outpatient counseling, others may find it necessary to transition to a sober living environment while undergoing outpatient treatment. For many in early recovery, maintaining sobriety is significantly enhanced when they are not immediately reintegrated into familiar environments or surrounded by the same people, places, and triggers they encountered prior to treatment.

With an epidemic of this magnitude, we need to initiate a massive, influential campaign to make a dramatic leap forward in the public's understanding of addiction and the treatments that are available. Social media has proven to be the most effective means by which to create such an elevation in human awareness and action.

ADDICTION IS A FAMILY DISEASE

Family and a positive support system play a crucial role in helping a person struggling with addiction. Providing a loving, non-enabling support structure for those with SUD can increase their chances for a long, sober life.

Sadly, addiction does not just affect those using drugs or alcohol but can cause upheaval and chaos in the lives of their loved ones. Family and friends can experience depression, anxiety, anger, and powerlessness as they face what appears to be an ongoing crisis.

And the problem is immense. The National Survey on Drug Use and Health (NSDUH) estimates that 19.7 million Americans (aged twelve and older) battled SUD in 2017, the last year statistics were available.[11] How many friends and family members do you think were affected by those nearly twenty million people?

The addicted person can be an all-consuming issue in a support person's life, as they endure countless sleepless and hellish nights, wondering where their loved one is or if they are even alive. Family and friends get stuck in a cycle of fixing and then grow resentful when this fix doesn't work or is not appreciated. Even worse is the guilt they can feel as their loved one sinks deeper and deeper into addiction or dies a tragic death.

Here is some helpful advice I suggest to families helping a loved one struggling with SUD.

#1: Education, education, education

When family members understand addiction and how much control it holds over someone with SUD, they tend to become more compassionate. By learning that addiction changes the brain in ways beyond a person's control, loved ones can adapt how they assist someone struggling with SUD.

I always recommend that close family members and caregivers consult a professional, such as a therapist specializing in addiction treatment. Additionally, Al-Anon is a free program that supports families of individuals with addiction. It provides a valuable opportunity for loved ones to learn from the experiences of others who have faced similar challenges. One of the Al-Anon program's

---

[11] Substance Abuse and Mental Health Services Administration (SAMHSA), "Key Substance Use and Mental Health Indicators in the United States: Results from the 2017 National Survey on Drug Use and Health." September 14, 2018. https://www.samhsa.gov/data/report/2017-nsduh-annual-national-report.

basic principles is that of anonymity. Meetings are confidential, and they do not disclose who attends. A simple Google search of Al-Anon will show where local meetings are being held, or you may call 888-425-2666 for more information. Patience is also critical as this disease tends to be a chronic struggle and one that isn't typically "fixed" quickly. Remember that relapses are common and do not mean that all previous progress has been lost.

#2: Get help yourself

Loved ones struggling with SUD can emotionally drain the entire family. Oftentimes, family members become so focused on helping the afflicted person that they neglect other siblings or their spouse and even forfeit self-care. The whole family has become sick; therefore, the whole family needs to get well. Family members need care and attention.

Family members often torture themselves with feelings of guilt, wondering if it was somehow their fault that their loved one became addicted to drugs or alcohol. Please know that addiction is not something you "caused." While this concept can certainly be difficult at first, please try to understand SUD the same as you would any other medical condition.

I advocate a routine of regular exercise, healthy eating, and sleep for family members. Since being around loved ones struggling with SUD can be quite draining physically and emotionally, make sure to do something healthy when you leave the house.

Seek mental health support where you can share your feelings in a safe, non-judgmental space, whether with a private therapist or in Al-Anon meetings. This provides a positive and necessary outlet for building strength and unity. Don't underestimate the value of learning from other families facing situations similar to yours.

#3: Encourage treatment

One of your biggest challenges in loving a person who has an addiction is helping that person understand they have an issue in the first place. People struggling with SUD are often reluctant to acknowledge that they have a problem despite failing to fulfill responsibilities, maintain relationships, and keep up with their jobs. Denial is a vicious way in which addiction captures the mind.

I recommend a heartfelt intervention, where a trained interventionist and the family gather around to help the person understand their self-destructive behavior. Randy Grimes is a former NFL player in recovery from an addiction to painkillers who now conducts interventions across the country. He outlines the process he uses for interventions in his book *Off Center*. His book might be a useful read to understand what an intervention involves and why you want the help of a trained professional instead of doing it on your own.

If the addicted person refuses to seek help, which unfortunately is often the case, family members may need to apply pressure using any leverage they have (such as financial support, divorce proceedings, custody arrangements, or employing "tough love"). This leverage can be crucial in prompting the addicted person to seriously consider treatment options.

A powerful adjunct would be to get the person with an addiction to accept at least one shot of Vivitrol or the long-acting injection of Suboxone (Sublocade) after treatment as an additional concession. Usually, a refusal to get one is an indicator that they have not committed to stop using.

#4: Take part in treatment

Some of the better inpatient rehabs and outpatient counseling centers require or strongly suggest family participation in treatment. Make sure to attend Family Days and ask your loved one to sign a release for you to be able to speak with their counselors and doctors.

I took part in the creation of the first-of-its-kind Vivitrol support group that started in Long Island, New York, in 2015. The Nassau County government at that time not only helped in the creation of this meeting, but also created a comprehensive "shot at life" program. This county program helped connect people with addiction to doctors who could help them get started with Vivitrol treatment. The Vivitrol support group was geared toward those who either wanted to learn about Vivitrol or were already receiving this treatment. This meeting was also open to family members who wanted to learn more about Vivitrol.

In many instances, the first person attending the Vivitrol group was a parent seeking help for their child suffering from SUD. Most were at their wits' end and were afraid of losing their loved ones to the deadly effects of SUD. One mother had two boxes full of the research she conducted in the hopes of rescuing her son. She was shocked to find that none of her work came up with Vivitrol as an option. When hearing about it, she attended the support group and now, literally, has her son back.

#5: Find the balance between support and enabling

Tim Ryan, author of *From Dope to Hope* and a nationally renowned recovery speaker, said to me recently: "If you baby them, you will bury them" in speaking about how families almost always enable the member who is addicted. Oftentimes, families try to wrongly support the person dealing with addiction by covering for them, lending them money, and picking up the slack. I advocate setting strict boundaries while maintaining a loving and supportive environment.

It is crucial that the person dealing with SUD feels that they can depend on their family, but they also need to feel the consequences of their actions. Family members should communicate clear boundaries and stay strong while the person dealing with SUD endures any negative consequences. Often, when someone is in the throes of addiction, the disease causes them to use emotional manipulation in order to obtain money for more drugs. While it can be devastating to have your loved one use this tactic, please try to remember that this is part of the disease for almost everyone, and it has very little to do with how they truly feel. Do not allow this maneuver to deceive you. Instead, stand firm and offer your loving support in ways that can help them but never in ways that can facilitate more drug use. For example, if they ask for grocery money, do not give cash but go shopping with them instead.

#6: Get trained to save a life

Most fatal overdoses happen in the comfort of people's homes. Whether your loved one is using heroin or legally prescribed opiate painkillers, there is always a risk that an overdose could occur. If, God forbid, you ever came upon someone who has had an overdose, it is possible to save their life—without any medical training.

Narcan (generic name = naloxone) is a nasal spray that can be easily administered within seconds. In the event of a potentially deadly overdose where a loved one is unconscious, a single spray of Narcan swiftly enters the brain, displacing opioids from their receptors and restoring breathing. Essentially, Narcan functions as a rapid and short-acting form of Vivitrol. While Narcan can save a person's life during an overdose, its effects typically last for no more than an hour. Therefore, while it can rescue someone from overdose, it is not for the ongoing treatment of addiction. Narcan can be obtained without a prescription at most major pharmacies across the country. As a standard practice for nearly all of my patients struggling with opioid addiction, I will prescribe Narcan to family members. This ensures they have it readily accessible at home in case of an emergency.

If you or a loved one is struggling with opioid addiction, it is absolutely imperative that you keep Narcan in your home and anywhere else that is essential. Countless lives have been saved from certain death because Narcan was administered in time.

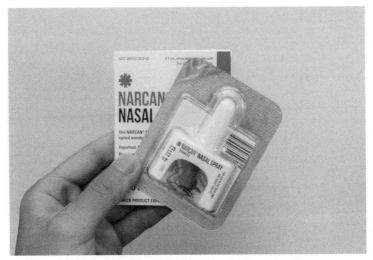

Narcan (naloxone) nasal spray: Now available over the counter at your local pharmacy without a prescription. This life-saving medication can be easily sprayed into the nose of someone over-dosing on opioids to quickly restore breathing and oxygen to the brain, potentially saving their life before the ambulance arrives. As a physician, I emphatically recommend that anyone strug-gling with addiction and their families keep naloxone at home.

#7: Clean up your own life

Begin at home. Remember how powerful environmental triggers can be in causing a relapse. Secure your alcohol and clean out your medicine cabinet. If visiting relatives, gently remind them to do the same.

Temptation leads to relapse. It is hard to be diplomatic in someone else's home about the dangers to your loved one with SUD, but it must be done. While in early recovery, your loved one is most vulnerable. A quiet word to the side can save much heartache later.

Setting an example is also a great way to show you care. It doesn't matter if the person who is in early recovery tells you that they are not triggered by watching you have a drink. Don't do it! That person may seem completely fine to you; heck, they might even believe that they are, but drinking or drugging in front of them will often light up their brain's limbic system on a subconscious level, which will manifest as conscious cravings for them over the next couple of days. So, please wait to drink when your loved one is not around. Show them that you too can be strong and forgo a glass of wine at dinner or a beer after work. Be the example you are asking them to be.

18

RECOVERY CROSSROADS: NAVIGATING MARIJUANA'S ROLE IN SOBRIETY

Marijuana (aka, cannabis or pot) was first used in Asian medicine around 500 BC. In the United States, we have a highly conflicted relationship with marijuana. Although it was outlawed in the United States by the federal Controlled Substance Act in 1970, many individual states have passed legislation to legalize marijuana use. Some have passed laws allowing marijuana to be used recreationally, while others have restricted its use only for specific medical conditions. In New York, where I practice medicine, "medical marijuana" was approved in 2018 for a limited set of specific medical conditions, one of which is to help with the treatment of opioid addiction. Fortunately, New York does have a requirement that medical marijuana, when used to help with opioid addiction, must be prescribed along with a comprehensive treatment program. In other words, that individual must be either enrolled or have completed an outpatient addiction treatment program.

To get medical marijuana in the state of New York, patients must first receive a prescription from a doctor who has been certified by the state to prescribe it. Regardless of their specialty, all doctors must obtain additional certification to prescribe medical marijuana. The physician enters the prescription into the state's online database and then provides the patient with a printed certification form. Prior to visiting the dispensary, patients are required to register online, entering their demographic information along with the number from their certification form. This process enables them to print an ID card. They can use their card at any number of medical marijuana dispensaries in the state, and they can select marijuana in many forms, including tinctures (droplets used under the tongue), smoking it with a vape device, and even different forms of edibles. The prescribing physician, however, can select restrictions on the prescription, including the concentration of tetrahydrocannabinol (THC) and the form of use.

It is beyond the scope of this book to discuss the risks/benefits of marijuana outside of its specific use for the treatment of opioid addiction. However, I would like to make the following important points. Extensive research has shown that marijuana use, especially high-potency products, is associated with various mental health issues including schizophrenia, anxiety, and depression. It is well understood that marijuana specifically affects brain development. Developing brains, such as those in babies, children, and teenagers, are especially susceptible to the harmful effects of marijuana.[12, 13] In the last few years, there have been several studies demonstrating a link between marijuana and psychosis as well. Additionally, it's important to note that marijuana use by mothers during pregnancy could be linked to problems with attention,

[12] National Academies of Sciences, Engineering, and Medicine. "The Health Effects of Cannabis and Cannabinoids: The Current State of Evidence and Recommendations for Research." Washington, DC: The National Academies Press, 2017. https://nap.nationalacademies.org/catalog/24625/the-health-effects-of-cannabis-and-cannabinoids-the-current-state.

[13] Batalla, Albert, Sagnik Bhattacharyya, Murat Yücel, et al. "Structural and Functional Imaging Studies in Chronic Cannabis Users: A Systematic Review of Adolescent and Adult Findings." *PloS One* 8, no. 2 (February 2013): e55821. https://journals.plos.org/plosone/article?id=10.1371/journal.pone.0055821.

memory, problem-solving skills, and behavior in their children.[14, 15, 16, 17, 18, 19]

Using marijuana before age eighteen may affect how the brain builds connections for functions like attention, memory, and learning.[20] Youth who use marijuana may not do as well in school

[14] Grewen, Karen, Andrew P. Salzwedel, and Wei Gao. "Functional Connectivity Disruption in Neonates with Prenatal Marijuana Exposure." *Frontiers in Human Neuroscience* 9 (November 2015): 601. https://www.ncbi.nlm.nih.gov/pmc/articles/PMC4631947/.

[15] Goldschmidt, L., N. L. Day, and G. A. Richardson. "Effects of prenatal marijuana exposure on child behavior problems at age 10." *Neurotoxicology and Teratology* 22, no. 3 (May–June 2000): 325–336. https://pubmed.ncbi.nlm.nih.gov/10840176/.

[16] Leech, S. L., G. A. Richardson, L. Goldschmidt, and N. L. Day. "Prenatal substance exposure: effects on attention and impulsivity of 6-year-olds." *Neurotoxicology and Teratology* 21, no. 2 (March–April 1999): 109–118. https://pubmed.ncbi.nlm.nih.gov/10192271/.

[17] Fried, P. A., B. Watkinson, and R. Gray. "Differential effects on cognitive functioning in 9- to 12-year-olds prenatally exposed to cigarettes and marihuana. *Neurotoxicology and Teratology* 20, no. 3 (May–June 1998): 293–306. https://pubmed.ncbi.nlm.nih.gov/9638687/.

[18] El Marroun, Hanan, James J. Hudziak, Henning Tiemeier, et al. "Intrauterine cannabis exposure leads to more aggressive behavior and attention problems in 18-month-old girls." *Drug and Alcohol Dependence* 118, no. 2–3 (November 2011): 470–474. https://pubmed.ncbi.nlm.nih.gov/21470799/.

[19] Ryan, Sheryl A., Seth D. Ammerman, and Mary E. O'Connor. "Marijuana Use During Pregnancy and Breastfeeding: Implications for Neonatal and Childhood Outcomes." *Pediatrics* 142, no. 3 (September 2018): e20181889. https://pubmed.ncbi.nlm.nih.gov/30150209/.

[20] S. Department of Health and Human Services. National Institutes of Health. National Institute on Drug Abuse. https://www.drugabuse.gov/drug-topics/marijuana.

and may have trouble remembering things.[21, 22, 23, 24] These effects may last a long time or even be permanent,[25] but more research is needed to fully understand these effects.

A recent study published in the prestigious journal of *Psychological Medicine* has revealed a startling finding: teenagers who use cannabis face an elevenfold increase in the risk of developing a psychotic disorder compared to non-users.

This study adds to the growing body of evidence linking cannabis use to heightened risks of psychotic disorders, particularly during adolescence. Interestingly, no such correlation was found between cannabis use and psychotic disorders among individuals who began smoking after the age of twenty.

There appears to be a critical period during brain development where cannabis use escalates the risk of psychosis. This study underscores the importance of delaying cannabis use until later in life, potentially mitigating one of its most severe risks.

Does marijuana actually help people struggling with opioid addiction? As you might have guessed, this topic is fraught with controversy. Marijuana is hailed as a "wonder drug" or, in contrast,

---

21 "The Health Effects of Cannabis and Cannabinoids."
22 Goldschmidt, "Effects of prenatal marijuana exposure on child behavior problems at age 10."
23 "The Health Effects of Cannabis and Cannabinoids."
24 Filbey, Francesca M., Sina Aslan, Vince D. Calhoun, et al. "Long-term effects of marijuana use on the brain." *Proceedings of the National Academy of Sciences* 111, no. 47 (November 2014): 16913–16918. https://pubmed.ncbi.nlm.nih.gov/25385625/.
25 Meier, Madeline H., Avshalom Caspi, Antony Ambler, et al. "Persistent cannabis users show neuropsychological decline from childhood to midlife." *Proceedings of the National Academy of Sciences* 109, no. 40 (October 2012): E2657–E2664. https://pubmed.ncbi.nlm.nih.gov/22927402/.

a "gateway drug," depending on which expert you ask. It is for this very reason that I thought it necessary to discuss in this book.

The truth is, like most treatments in medicine, one size doesn't fit all. How someone feels and how marijuana affects their brain can vary greatly based on their unique neural makeup. Some individuals may experience heightened anxiety, paranoia, or even panic attacks when using marijuana. Conversely, others may feel more creative, focused, relaxed, or energized. For certain individuals who have managed to get sober from opioid drugs, the option of using marijuana intermittently to calm down drug cravings and prevent relapse is very helpful. However, this is not the case for everyone. For some people in sobriety, using marijuana can actually trigger cravings for their true drug of choice (opioids). This is a further demonstration of how addiction is not just about the drug itself but just as much about the individual's brain and how the two interact. In other words, how a particular drug affects a person's limbic system is different from person to person. Not everyone is affected the same.

A final point to remember: CBD (cannabidiol) should not be confused with marijuana, even though they're often mentioned together. Marijuana contains both CBD and THC, but only THC induces intoxication or euphoria (the "high"). THC is also the component that, in some cases, helps to treat opioid addiction. Simply put, products containing only CBD do not have mood-altering or addictive effects and are generally not effective in treating addiction. There has been some recent research suggesting that CBD can be helpful for certain specific medical conditions, such as epilepsy. In 2018, the FDA approved the drug Epidiolex, a pharmaceutical-grade strain of CBD, for the treatment of certain forms of epilepsy. However, the vast majority of people who take CBD are not using it for this purpose. In fact, it's likely that you've already come across "CBD" prominently displayed on the shelves of your local grocery store or vitamin shop. It's being advertised to help with anxiety, stress, insomnia, and many other conditions. It's sold in numerous different forms—everything from delicious chocolates to dog treats. CBD is also offered in various different topical creams to help with your aching joints and muscles. It's important to remember though that while CBD is considered safe, there is essentially no good evidence to support any of these claims.

In summary, there is some evidence to support the use of medical marijuana to help people with their recovery from opiate addiction. However, this won't help everyone trying to stay sober, and in fact, for some, it can actually be harmful. To minimize this risk, marijuana for this purpose should always be under the direction of a physician and used in the setting of a comprehensive opioid addiction treatment program that involves ongoing counseling.

TELEMEDICINE: THE NEW FRONTIER

The pandemic lockdowns of 2020 have devastated those suffering with mental illness and addiction. I agree with the many other experts who have said that the lockdowns have led to more suffering and death than the COVID-19 virus itself. In fact, a study out of Johns Hopkins showed that the lockdowns offered no benefit to society whatsoever.[26] The forced isolation has seen the number of fatal drug overdoses and suicide attempts skyrocket, along with alcohol consumption increasing tremendously. The closing of churches (where 12-step meetings are often held), job losses, financial instability, and the closure of gyms have taken away vital aspects of those in recovery.

---

[26] Herby, Jonas, Lars Jonung, and Steve H. Hanke. "A Literature Review and Meta-Analysis of the Effects of Lockdowns on Covid-19 Mortality," *Studies in Applied Economics*, no. 200 (January 2022). https://sites.krieger.jhu.edu/iae/files/2022/01/A-Literature-Review-and-Meta-Analysis-of-the-Effects-of-Lockdowns-on-COVID-19-Mortality.pdf.

Missed medical care has been another terrible consequence. Roughly half the American population did not show up for their cancer screenings. These cancers did not just go away but will now be detected at a later stage and in a more advanced form. It's been estimated that roughly half of chemotherapy appointments in this country were missed due to fear of leaving home.

Thankfully, one enormously positive benefit that came out of lockdowns was the rapid expansion of telehealth. Telehealth has allowed doctors of all specialties to consult with patients from their homes.

Telehealth, also known as telemedicine, connects our most vulnerable populations with services they might not otherwise have received and has greatly expanded access to medical and psychiatric care. Federal and state governments have also stepped in, mandating that insurance companies cover telemedicine visits.

Telehealth has given us the ability to provide care for people across the country, especially in rural areas where there are few mental health practitioners and even fewer addiction specialists. With a simple cell phone, someone can connect to doctors on demand all over the world. Using various face-to-face apps available, doctors can literally see their patients and are able to extrapolate information about their condition in better ways than purely by voice interpretation.

While telehealth had been available even prior to the COVID-19 pandemic, there were many legal and insurance reimbursement issues that hindered its ability to be used. For example, many insurance companies wouldn't reimburse for telehealth appointments if the patient was in their own home during the time of the consultation. Instead, it required that the person visit a local doctor's office or designated medical center and then perform the telemedicine appointment from that facility. Also, physicians were unable to treat patients if they resided in a state where that physician did not have a license to practice medicine. During the pandemic, most states dropped these regulations and allowed physicians licensed in any state to see patients who resided in any other state. During this time, I provided care to hundreds of individuals located across the United States, particularly in very rural areas. Unfortunately, many states have now begun to roll back these expanded privileges for doctors to see patients outside their state. I am extremely concerned about this as it could leave many individuals, particularly those in remote areas, without access to their doctors and medications.

A recent large-scale poll conducted by the Harris Poll in conjunction with Alkermes, the maker of Vivitrol, revealed that patients have shown extremely high satisfaction with telehealth. One in four people currently use telepsychiatry for mental health care, with over 70 percent expressing a favorable impression. Sixty percent indicated that they could not have received the care they needed without it, and 75 percent expressed interest in continuing telehealth even after the COVID-19 restrictions are lifted.

It is likely that many individuals who need treatment for mental health, and particularly for addiction, are not comfortable going to a psychiatrist's office or an addiction treatment center because of the stigma. A higher percentage of patients appear to be keeping their appointments when it can be done via telehealth. Telehealth also eliminates travel barriers for the indigent and reduces the risk of exposure to illness while on public transportation.

In 2020, I started bringing addiction and mental health services to people in a rural New York county through telehealth. Each week I dedicated time to seeing patients suffering with SUD and mental health conditions via telehealth in Sullivan County, New York. This region of the state has high levels of poverty, mental illness, and drug addiction, paired with very few physicians who specialize in mental health and even fewer trained in addiction. Like many other regions in the country, fatal overdoses continue to climb from the opiate addiction crisis with very little access to help.

Leaders in Sullivan County asked me to not only help treat their patients via telehealth but also teach their local psychiatrists about addiction and the latest MAT protocols. Prior to this, the county's physicians had yet to treat even one single patient addicted to opiates with Vivitrol. Together, we have developed a telehealth model for their county that I believe will soon be used as a model for the rest of the nation.

Unfortunately, not enough people are aware that telehealth services exist or know how to access them. I urge all physicians and mental health/addiction counselors to offer telemedicine to their patients with great urgency. The public must become aware of telehealth and learn how to access it.

This country's addiction and mental health system is vastly underfunded and fragmented. I urge national media and insurance companies to launch a campaign to increase public awareness about the availability of telehealth and how easily it can be utilized. Telehealth is going to play a very large role in the future of addiction medicine. It is an idea whose time has come.

THE BLUEPRINT FOR HEALING

Opioid addiction is a medical emergency! Every single time that someone uses opioid drugs they are quite literally putting their life on the line. It's not a matter of if but when a person actively using opioids will overdose and die. Remember that a person in the throes of opioid addiction will be seeking out and using the drug every single day. With fentanyl now mixed into every sample of opioids, how much longer can you or your loved one survive? You must take action immediately!

If you or a loved one are grappling with addiction and unsure where to turn for assistance, reach out to SAMHSA (Substance Abuse and Mental Health Services Administration). SAMHSA's National Helpline at 1-800-662-4357 is a confidential, free, 24/7 information service available in English and Spanish for individuals and families dealing with mental health and/or substance use disorders. This service offers referrals to local treatment facilities, support groups, and community-based organizations.

You can also find help near you by visiting the online treatment locator at www.findtreatment.gov or by texting your zip code to 435748 (HELP4U). Be honest about what you are going through. Become informed about the medication and counseling options available. And don't allow yourself to believe that you are destined to end up in prison or dead. Regardless of how many relapses or treatment programs you've been through, you are always capable of achieving prolonged recovery and living your best life.

As I penned these words, my primary aim was to convey to you the very same life-saving information that I've had the privilege of sharing with addiction doctors throughout America. This book is not merely a compilation of facts and insights; it's a beacon of hope and the key to recovery.

With the newfound awareness you gain from reading these pages, you also inherit a significant responsibility. It's not enough to keep this knowledge to yourself; it's imperative to share it with those who might be in desperate need of guidance and support. Your actions today have the potential to ripple through time, positively impacting the lives of countless individuals tomorrow.

Every person you encounter, whether a friend, family member, colleague, or stranger, is in the battle of their life or is intimately connected to someone who is. It's crucial to recognize this shared humanity and extend a helping hand whenever possible. By sharing this vital information, you have the power to offer hope, healing, and a path toward recovery to those who may feel lost or alone.

So, I implore you: do not underestimate the significance of your words, your actions, or even your thoughts. What may seem like a simple gesture or passing conversation could be the lifeline that someone desperately needs. Reach out, speak up, and spread the message of hope and healing far and wide.

In doing so, you become a catalyst for change, a beacon of light in the darkness of addiction. Thank you for joining me on this journey. Together, we can change lives and build a world where compassion, understanding, and support prevail.

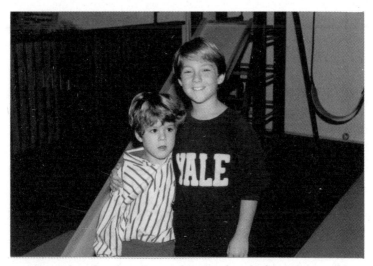

Me and my brother, Travis, sharing a bond of pure love and joy. Our relationship was marked by unwavering support and affection. Even as we faced his struggles, my love for him was constant and boundless. This photo captures the incredible closeness of our bond, a testament to the enduring love that continues to inspire and guide me in my work and life.

REFERENCES

Adolescent Brain Cognitive Development. https://abcdstudy. org/.

"AG James, States Reach Settlement with Reckitt over Allegations of Improper Marketing of Suboxone," press release, October 23, 2019, https://ag.ny.gov/press-release/2019/ ag-james-states-reach-settlement-reckitt-over-allegations-improper-marketing.

"Alkermes Responds to Senator's Inquiry," press release, November 6, 2017, http://media.corporate-ir.net/media_files/ IROL/92/92211/Alkermes Responds to Senator%E2%80 %99s Inquiry.pdf.

Batalla, Albert, Sagnik Bhattacharyya, Murat Yücel, et al. "Structural and Functional Imaging Studies in Chronic Cannabis Users: A Systematic Review of Adolescent and Adult Findings." *PloS One* 8, no. 2 (February 2013):e55821. https:// journals.plos.org/plosone/article?id=10.1371/journal. pone.0055821.

Botticelli, Michael. "Why Trump's opioid plan falls short." STAT. March 20, 2018. https://www.statnews.com/2018/03/20/ trump-opioid-plan/.

Centers for Disease Control and Prevention (CDC). "Provisional Drug Overdose Death Counts." https://www.cdc.gov/nchs/nvss/vsrr/drug-overdose-data.htm#:~:-text=1%3B%20natural%20and%20semisynthetic%20opioids,4%3B%20cocaine%2C%20T40.

Dean, Angela J., John B. Saunders, Rod T. Jones, et al. "Does naltrexone treatment lead to depression? Findings from a randomized controlled trial in subjects with opioid dependence." *Journal of Psychiatry and Neuroscience* 31, no. 1 (January 2006): 38–45. https://www.ncbi.nlm.nih.gov/pmc/articles/PMC1325065/#:~:text=In%20the%20subset%20of%20subjects,with%20those%20on%20methadone%20maintenance.

El Marroun, Hanan, James J. Hudziak, Henning Tiemeier, et al. "Intrauterine cannabis exposure leads to more aggressive behavior and attention problems in 18-month-old girls." *Drug and Alcohol Dependence* 118, no. 2–3 (November 2011): 470–474. https://pubmed.ncbi.nlm.nih.gov/21470799/.

Filbey, Francesca M., Sina Aslan, Vince D. Calhoun, et al. "Long-term effects of marijuana use on the brain." *Proceedings of the National Academy of Sciences* 111, no. 47 (November 2014): 16913–16918. https://pubmed.ncbi.nlm.nih.gov/25385625/.

Fried, P. A., B. Watkinson, and R. Gray. "Differential effects on cognitive functioning in 9- to 12-year-olds prenatally exposed to cigarettes and marihuana. *Neurotoxicology and Teratology* 20, no. 3 (May–June 1998): 293–306. https://pubmed.ncbi.nlm.nih.gov/9638687/.

Goldschmidt, L., N. L. Day, and G. A. Richardson. "Effects of prenatal marijuana exposure on child behavior problems at age 10." *Neurotoxicology and Teratology* 22, no. 3 (May–June 2000): 325–336. https://pubmed.ncbi.nlm.nih.gov/10840176/.

Grewen, Karen, Andrew P. Salzwedel, and Wei Gao. "Functional Connectivity Disruption in Neonates with Prenatal Marijuana Exposure." *Frontiers in Human Neuroscience* 9 (November 2015): 601. https://www.ncbi.nlm.nih.gov/pmc/articles/PMC4631947/.

Herby, Jonas, Lars Jonung, and Steve H. Hanke, "A Literature Review and Meta-Analysis of the Effects of Lockdowns on Covid-19 Mortality." *Studies in Applied Economics*, no. 200 (January 2022). https://sites.krieger.jhu.edu/iae/files/2022/01/A-Literature-Review-and-Meta-Analysis-of-the-Effects-of-Lockdowns-on-COVID-19-Mortality.pdf.

Krupitsky, Evgeny, Edward V. Nunes, Walter Ling, et al. "Injectable extended-release naltrexone for opioid dependence: a double-blind, placebo-controlled, multicentre randomised trial." *The Lancet* 377, no. 9776 (April 2011): 1506–1513. https://pubmed.ncbi.nlm.nih.gov/21529928/.

Leech, S. L., G. A. Richardson, L. Goldschmidt, and N. L. Day. "Prenatal substance exposure: effects on attention and impulsivity of 6-year-olds." *Neurotoxicology and Teratology* 21, no. 2 (March–April 1999): 109–118. https://pubmed.ncbi.nlm.nih.gov/10192271/.

Lee, MD, Dr. Joshua D., Edward V. Nunes Jr., MD, Patricia Novo, MPH, et al. "Comparative effectiveness of extended-release naltrexone versus buprenorphine-naloxone for opioid relapse prevention." *The Lancet* 391, no. 10118 (November 2017): 309–318, https://www.thelancet.com/journals/lancet/article/PIIS0140-6736(17)32812-X/fulltext.

Meier, Madeline H., Avshalom Caspi, Antony Ambler, et al. "Persistent cannabis users show neuropsychological decline from childhood to midlife." *Proceedings of the National Academy of Sciences* 109, no. 40 (October 2012): E2657–E2664. https://pubmed.ncbi.nlm.nih.gov/22927402/.

National Academies of Sciences, Engineering, and Medicine. "The Health Effects of Cannabis and Cannabinoids: The Current State of Evidence and Recommendations for Research." Washington, DC: The National Academies Press, 2017. https://nap.nationalacademies.org/catalog/24625/the-health-effects-of-cannabis-and-cannabinoids-the-current-state.

Ralston, Meghan. "The End of the Addict." *Drug Policy Alliance.* March 23, 2014. drugpolicy.org/blog/end-addict.

Ryan, Sheryl A., Seth D. Ammerman, and Mary E. O'Connor. "Marijuana Use During Pregnancy and Breastfeeding: Implications for Neonatal and Childhood Outcomes." *Pediatrics* 142, no. 3 (September 2018): e20181889. https://pubmed.ncbi.nlm.nih.gov/30150209/.

Tanum, Lars, Kristin Klemmetsby Solli, Zill-E-Huma Latif, et al. "Effectiveness of Injectable Extended-Release Naltrexone vs Daily Buprenorphine-Naloxone for Opioid Dependence: A Randomized Clinical Noninferiority Trial." *JAMA Psychiatry* 74, no. 12 (December 2017): 1197–1205. doi:10.1001/jamapsychiatry.2017.3206.

"Telehealth: The Coming 'New Normal' for Healthcare." The Harris Poll. May 11, 2020. https://theharrispoll.com/briefs/telehealth-new-normal-healthcare/.

S. Department of Health and Human Services. National Institutes of Health. National Institute on Drug Abuse. https://www.drugabuse.gov/drug-topics/marijuana.

Substance Abuse and Mental Health Services Administration (SAMHSA), "Key Substance Use and Mental Health Indicators in the United States: Results from the 2017 National Survey on Drug Use and Health." September 14, 2018. https://www.samhsa.gov/data/report/2017-nsduh-annual-national-report.

ABOUT THE AUTHOR

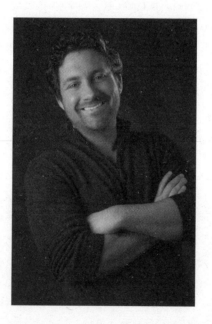

D r. Russell Surasky received his medical degree from the New York College of Osteopathic Medicine in 2009, receiving honors in multiple specialties, including psychiatry, family practice, and surgery. He completed his internship in internal medicine at Mount Sinai Queens Hospital Center in 2010 and his residency in neurology at North Shore University Hospital in 2013.

Dr. Surasky continues to receive national acclaim for his innovative and highly successful addiction treatment protocols. His advanced approach has helped thousands of patients rapidly achieve and sustain sobriety and has made Dr. Surasky among the most sought-after addiction specialists in the country.

Dr. Surasky regularly appears as a medical contributor on major news networks. Most recently, he has made several appearances on Fox News with Tucker Carlson and anchor Neil Cavuto. From the start of the COVID-19 pandemic, Dr. Surasky has been outspoken and highly critical of the pandemic lockdowns due to their overwhelmingly negative impact on mental health and the addiction crisis.

Dr. Surasky has spent many years acting as the medical director of a large multi-center drug addiction treatment program with multiple centers across New York. Additionally, he has been a national speaker on the topic of substance use disorders, educating physicians and the US criminal justice system about addiction and the latest advancements in treatment. He has also spearheaded a telehealth initiative to help bring addiction and mental health care to people living in rural and remote regions of the country. Most recently, Dr. Surasky has accepted a clinical and professorship role with one of the largest hospital systems in New York.

Dr. Surasky is the most experienced doctor in New York State utilizing Vivitrol, an incredibly effective and non-habit-forming medicine for the treatment of both opiate and alcohol use disorders.

Dr. Surasky maintains hospital privileges at North Shore University Hospitals of Manhasset, Plainview, and Syosset, New York, as well as Long Island Jewish Medical Center in New Hyde

Park, New York. He is actively involved in the medical community and is a member of several professional organizations, including the American Academy of Neurology, the American Society of Addiction Medicine, and the Nassau County Medical Society.